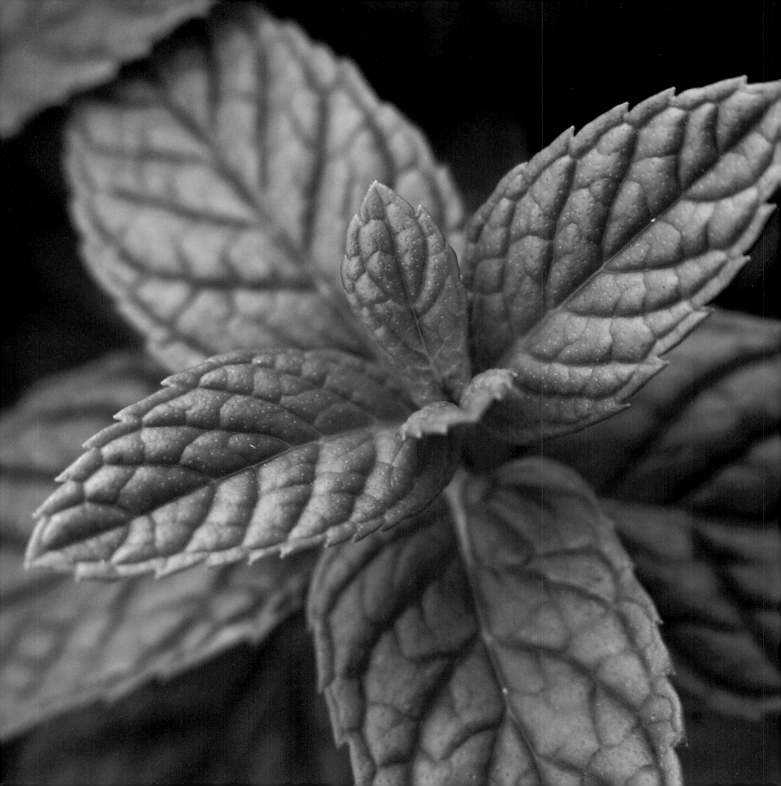

Essential Oils: A Beginner's Guide

Healthcare for Today

by Carrie Donegan & Elena Yordán

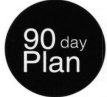

90 day **Plan**

Essential Oils: Healthcare for Today

A Beginner's Guide

Copyright © 2013 Diamond Circle. All rights reserved.

Published ISBN: 978-1-937702-13-7

First printing 2013

Published and Distributed by AromaTools

1351 West 800 North

Orem, UT 84057

Phone: 866-728-0070 or 801-798-7921

www.AromaTools.com

Email: service@AromaTools.com

God has created me to do Him some definite service; He has committed some work to me which He has not committed to another. I have my mission—I may never know it in this life, but I shall be told it in the next…I have a part in a great work; I am a link in a chain, a bond of connection between persons…

—Cardinal John Henry Newman

Our Mission

Most books on essential oils are written by doctors, scientists, nurses, healers, or religious leaders who have studied plants and their medicinal uses through the eye of a microscope or the eyes of their patients. Our humble testimony here is just that—a body of experience compiled for more than a decade and from the combined experiences of the thousands of people who have joined us in our quest for healthcare answers through self-care and natural solutions.

What we bring to you here is a beginning—a place to start. For each issue we have shared a possible use of essential oils and products. Are there more combinations? Of course; an unlimited number, in fact. But the question that one always asks at the beginning is, "Where do I start?"

We suggest you start here—*Essential Oils: Healthcare for Today.* Our simple guide, herein called the **Cheat Sheet,** will give you *the 90-Day Plan*, separated into 3 months, for each health issue presented. The information we provide is what has worked for us in our everyday lives and in those of our friends and families as well. We hope this guide will serve you as well as it has served us.

Let's keep the conversation going. Find us online at www.CarrieAndElena.com.

TOC

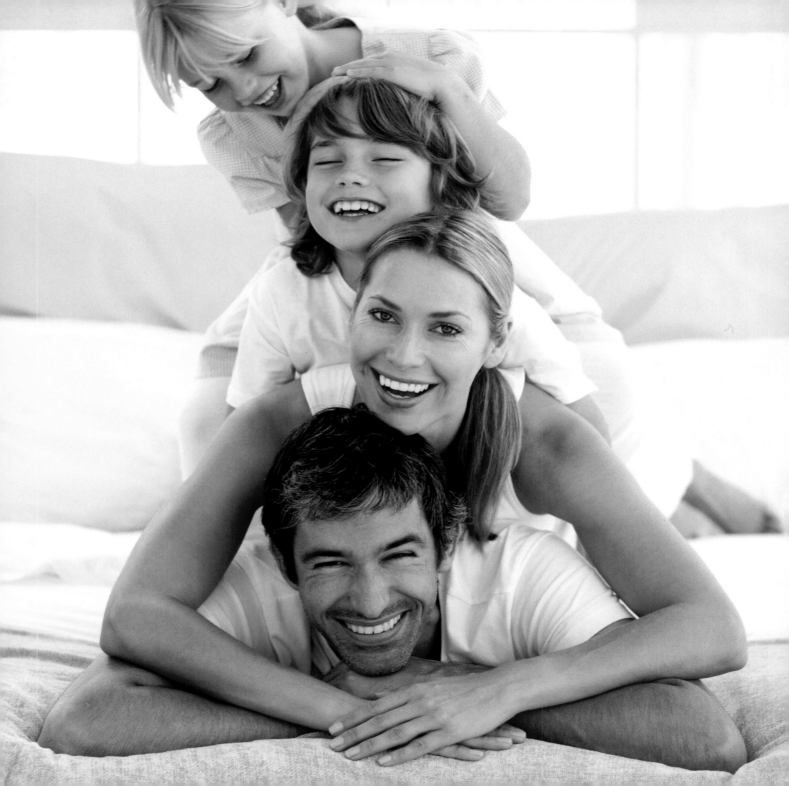

Acknowledgements

In many ways this book not only represents our experiences with essential oils and natural products but also represents a gathering of people: the community we came from, and the one that grew out of our search for information. There have been hundreds of meetings, meals, phone conversations, courses, lectures, conferences, and talks from which we have learned. There are also the thousands of people, across several continents, who have truly touched our lives and whom we value immeasurably. We bless them all for what they have done to help us.

As in any experience, there are people who are indispensable. The ones who stand by you, put up with your bad days, bandage your wounds, cheer you on, and pray for you. The following are those special people:

Our husbands and children: you made this book possible! You are our core, a constant source of love and inspiration. We are so grateful to: Fred, Carrie's husband, and their children, Rick & Ciara; José, Elena's husband, and their children, Laura & Henry. Our parents: we are both only children, raised by strong mothers, Sally Turner and Clara Ostrowski, who gave us a solid foundation, a strong faith formation, and an unwavering belief that we could do anything that we set out to do and to never waste the gifts we have been given. Bruce Turner, Carrie's step-dad and overall guardian angel to both of us. To our fathers, both gone too soon, we wish you could have been here to share this second book with us too.

Our friends and colleagues: Natalie Amoia, Lillian Brenwasser, Sonila Chaudry, Greg Cook, Judy Donegan, Paul Donegan, Donna Dillion, Mary Ann Durante, Christine Gehres, John Guarnieri & Lorinda Walker, Claudia Hanlin, Justin Harrison, Dr. David Hill, Mary Heffel, Bill & Laura Hemmer, Hong Leong Chua & Shu Li Law, Margarete Hyer, Jan Jeremias, Karin Johnson, Nick Killpack, Gerhard & Petra Krauss, Eric Larsen, Corey Lindley, Mitch Mensch, Gina McConeghy, Jennifer Minicus and our friends from Circle, Maria Morocho, Rochelle Olson, Todd Purser, Guitty Roustai & James Klein, Orly Rumberg, Sue Schultz, Jeff & Denise Schwendeman, René Spalek, David Stirling, Kerry Stonehouse, Cindy Tharayil, Lisa Ullman, Irene Weinberg, Rob Wilson, Emily Wright, and Rob Young.

Our followers on Facebook & Twitter: thank you for spreading the word! We could not have done this without you. We love and thank you all. In good health and deepest gratitude,

—Carrie & Elena

Introduction

Many people use essential oils—young and old alike. Before beginning this or any nutritional or exercise regimen, consult your physician to be sure it is appropriate for you. To use your oils as safely as possible, please follow the guidelines below.

Essential oil and product guidelines:

1. Always consult a medical professional before you incorporate essential oils and supplements into your health regimen.

2. Never put an oil directly into the eyes or the ears. If you do get an essential oil into the eyes or ears, do not panic. Apply *coconut oil* with a soft cloth, and gently wipe the essential oil out of the eyes. Within moments you should feel relief. If you have dripped an essential oil into the ear, you may pour a half teaspoon or less of *coconut oil* into the ear and then tip the head to pour it out. This should remove any discomfort to the ear.

3. We have come to prefer and trust therapeutic-grade products. We believe that oils which are not safe enough to ingest should not be diffused into the air or applied to the skin.

4. When applying oils to the skin for the first time, always dilute them. Some oils are generally regarded as mild enough to apply neat—directly to the skin, undiluted. However, if you have sensitive skin or for young children, always dilute the oil with *coconut oil* before applying.

5. Do not mix essential oils with synthetic personal care products, preservatives, or adulterated foods.

6. Keep bottles closed, out of direct light and high heat, so that your oils remain potent and long-lasting.

7. Keep essential oils out of reach of small children.

8. Pregnant women should always use essential oils only under the advisement of a medical professional.

Now that you know how to use essential oils safely, how do you begin?

This book, *Essential Oils: Healthcare for Today*, is a beginner's guide to health and business basics with essential oils. Here we have chosen products that we feel will help you get started using and sharing essential oils and products both quickly and easily. Once you have started, you may want to learn more; so we've also provided you with health tips (The Health Edit), studies (Your Inner Geek), resources (Dive In!), and our personal experiences (Integrate).

The 90-Day Plan was developed as both a guide for the beginning user and as a tool for the business builder. These plans are found in the *Cheat Sheets*, books, radio show, professional coaching program, websites, and our other marketing materials (go to **www.CarrieAndElena.com**). The *Cheat Sheets* are an easy way to help you improve your health in 90 days using essential oils and essential oil–based products. Information can also be found on Twitter, Facebook, and other social media. These are just some of the resources we provide to help you set out on the road to excellent, natural health. Stay tuned—there's more to come!

Open the bottle; feel a difference:

1. Pick one of the 50 health challenges listed here in *Essential Oils: Healthcare for Today*. Addressing too many issues at once is more difficult than dealing with them one at a time.

2. Look at the 90-Day Plan **Cheat Sheet** for each challenge. Order the products listed, and commit to using them for at least 90 days. Try to use up each order completely each month to get the best results.

3. The smartest way to order the products you love is through a monthly autoship program. These programs often provide free product credits for monthly purchases ordered through the program. Members of these programs can often earn rebates, bonuses, discounted shipping, and special offers. Take advantage of what is available.

4. The **Our Approach** section will show you how to use essential oils and essential oil products in three ways: **Apply** (applying to the skin), **Try** (dropping right on or under the tongue, in capsules, in water or tea, on a spoon with honey, or in food), and **Diffuse** (diffusing into the air through a small device or even into a cup of hot water or on a cotton ball).

5. Share your results with others. See our tips in the "Spread the word!" section below.

6. Keep using your oils and supplements for daily support and as challenges arise. Carry your oils with you and/or put them where you are most likely to see and use them everyday. Always have samples and materials on hand to share with others. *Don't forget to open a bottle and share!*

Spread the word!

When you find something that really works, your first instinct is to spread the word…a great restaurant, movie, or beautiful store! We are programmed to pass things on. This sounds like an easy thing to do, but some of us find talking to others challenging or even debilitating. Do I know enough to start talking to others? What should I say? Will people like what I have to say? What if I don't communicate well? What if I forget something? Sometimes these questions alone can stop us from helping a family member or friend who may be in need.

Introduction

Secrets for Success

Essential Oils: Healthcare for Today with its **90-Day Plan Cheat Sheets** is the perfect tool to spread the word about essential oils.

How do we know it will work for you? In 2007, we teamed up to achieve our goals because we knew that partnership and combining strengths was the key to success for any business. Elena came to the partnership with a business background in finance and entrepreneurship. Carrie added her experience in management and education.

While it was our passion for natural health that became the glue for our ideas, we each came to essential oils and supplements via different paths. In 2005, Carrie lost her hearing; and in 2007, Elena battled viral pneumonia with her 2 kids. Essential oil-based products brought both of them out of these challenges and into greater health.

For almost 2 years, we worked hard to find the best way to share essential oils with others. Although we tried many paths, one way kept rising to the top as the most successful: address one issue at a time, and work at it for 90 days. The concept of a 90-day plan is well known in business circles, and putting it together with health proved to be easy and effective.

By 2009, we had taken this concept to the next level by creating a business brand concept found in the *Cheat Sheet*. This brand concept builds on one simple idea in 3 easy steps:

1. Identify a need, and provide a solution.

2. Stick to it for 90 days.

3. Coach others to their own success.

The plan has been so successful that is now published in several languages, including English, Spanish, and German. This 90-Day Plan has also been featured on numerous blogs, websites, and other media outlets.

Most importantly, the 90-Day Plan works—both in theory and in practice. We have been able to reach the highest sales ranks in multiple essential oil companies and have helped countless others to do the same.

So, will it work for you? We believe it will! You don't need to remember or know anything special to be successful. The tools in this book will do the work for you. You can give this book to anyone interested in essential oils. The information inside will help them try something new, apply oils to new and old situations, and give them the success story they need to begin spreading the word themselves!

Once you have the right tools, it's easier to spread the word about essential oils and natural products. This book, *Essential Oils: Healthcare for Today,* with its 90-Day Plans will help you learn more and connect with others.

Follow these easy steps:

1. Carry a few copies of *Essential Oils: Healthcare for Today*, and pass them on to members of your team and to those you meet.

2. Plan ahead. Look at least 3 months out. Carry product samples and the booklet *Introduction to Modern Essentials* (available at www.aromatools.com), and put your contact information on them. Make it a personal goal to hand out at least two samples with information per day. Ask the person you give the sample to for their contact information so you can follow up in a few days. Follow up with 3 easy questions: Did you like it? Did it help? Would you like to get some more? You can help them get healthier and be in service to others.

3. Hold a 90-Day Plan meeting based on one of the fifty topics in this book. Give each person a small product sample, and have them follow the Plan on the **Cheat Sheet** for 90 days. You don't need to over-talk, over-explain, provide too much "science," or argue with naysayers! Listening well works wonders.

4. Go to www.CarrieAndElena.com, and send others there too. On this website are links to the *Dollars & Scents* radio show, blog, information on upcoming events, coaching, and more. You can sign up for Facebook and "LIKE" our page at www.facebook.com/CarrieAndElena to join our growing community of other essential oil users who love sharing information.

Thanks for reading, and here's to your good health!

— Carrie & Elena

Suggested Reading:

Making the First Circle Work by Randy Gage (Paperback, 2010).

One Minute Manager by Kenneth Blanchard & Spencer Johnson (Hardcover, 2003).

Permission Marketing: Turning Strangers Into Friends And Friends Into Customers by Seth Godin (Hardcover, 1999).

Delivering Happiness: A Path to Profits, Passion, and Purpose by Tony Hsieh (Hardcover, 2013).

Essential Oils Business Book: How to Start, Build, and Prosper in the Essential Oil Industry by Christina Calisto- Winslow (Paperback, 2010).

The Entrepreneur Equation: Evaluating the Realities, Risks, and Rewards of Having Your Own Business by Carol Roth (Paperback, 2012).

The Millionaire Next Door by Thomas J. Stanley and William D. Danko (Paperback, 1998) .

The Slight Edge by Jeff Olson (Paperback, 2011).

Addiction & Substance Abuse

Addiction is a physical or psychological dependence on something over which you feel you have no control. Many substances cross the blood-brain barrier, altering the chemical environment of the brain.

Our Approach

APPLY 2–4 drops of *cilantro* and *juniper* neat (undiluted) over the liver and on the bottoms of the feet 2 times daily. Drink plenty of water while using your oils to flush toxins from the body.

TRY 1 drop of *clove* and 1 drop of *black pepper* on the tip of the tongue every time a craving occurs. *Peppermint* has been known to help reduce food addictions when used frequently throughout the day (1 drop every 2 hours; or try a *Peppermint Beadlet*). Adding *Digestive Enzyme Complex* may help increase the absorption of nutrients that may be lacking in those who suffer from addictions. Improving your nutrition may also help you to overcome addictions.

CLEANSING is core to addiction cessation. Start with *GI Cleansing Formula,* and use it for 10 days. Then, incorporate *Detoxification Complex* capsules for 30 days. Remember, cleansing is an ongoing process and should be continued on a regular basis. Use *Digestive Blend* periodically to support healthy digestion.

DIFFUSE *peppermint* or *Joyful Blend* to change the chemical environment of your brain so that you can maintain your sobriety.

Your Inner Geek

In a review of research published in *Contemporary Nurse* in 2008, "The inhalation of essential oils acts on the central nervous system by… decreasing sympathetic nervous system activity and arousal of the autonomic nervous system," which can help to ease the tension associated with trying to end an addiction.

A controlled study by Rose & Behm in 1994 suggests that "inhalation of black pepper vapor may reduce the craving for cigarettes. In this trial, a total of 48 smokers used cigarette substitute devices that delivered black pepper vapor, menthol, or no fragrance. The results showed that use of the black pepper–based dummy cigarette reduced symptoms of craving for the first morning cigarette. Inhalation of vapor from black pepper extract reduces smoking withdrawal symptoms."
Drug Alcohol Dependence

> **Blessed is the man who remains steadfast under trial.**
> **—James 1:12**

Integrate

If you suffer from depression in addition to an addiction, your struggle may be much harder. Dealing with the depression can unlock the strength you need to overcome your addictions. Going on depression medications can lead to other addictions and may not be the most desirable course. Try following the 90-Day Plan Cheat Sheet for Depression. This plan can be used by all, regardless of age, and includes nutritional and essential oil suggestions.

Did you know?

According to goop.com's "How to Break a Habit…or Start a New One," habits are much more powerful than we realize. So often we act out of what we are used to, what we know, or what we have done in the past instead of making a better choice—a choice in the moment that might be for our higher good. They note that oftentimes detrimental behaviors can be modified by focusing on changing patterns and forming new neural pathways.

Dive In!

Making Habits, Breaking Habits: Why We Do Things, Why We Don't, and How to Make Any Change Stick by Jeremy Dean (Hardcover 2013).

"The Power of Habit" by Charles Duhigg, *The New York Times*, March 9, 2012.

GetSomeHeadspace.com by Andy Puddicombe.

"DrugFacts: High School and Youth Trends" *National Institute on Drug Abuse*, drugabuse.gov, December 2012.

Cheat Sheet

MONTH 1
black pepper
cilantro
GI Cleansing Formula
peppermint
Detoxification Complex

MONTH 2
black pepper
clove
Joyful Blend
Juniper
Digestive Complex

MONTH 3
black pepper
Digestive Blend
peppermint
Digestive Complex

90 day Plan

"Remember, you don't ever break a habit. If you want to get rid of bad behavior, you have to replace it with something positive, something that will make you stronger instead of weaker. Work on identifying positive behaviors that would make good replacements for your addictions."
—Dr. Phil McGraw

Allergies

An allergy is a damaging immune response by the body and can have many diverse causes, including hay fever, seasonal changes, poison ivy or other plants, molds, foods, animals, insect bites, drugs, cosmetics, or cleaners.

 ## Our Approach

APPLY *eucalyptus* or *Respiratory Blend* (dilute for young or sensitive skin) along the sides of the nose, on the throat, and on the back of the neck to help relieve symptoms. Apply **Calming Blend** neat around a rash to soothe the itch.

TRY *Daily Supplements Pack* with a capsule of *lavender* (start with 1 drop; increase if needed; 2–4 times a day). Add 1–2 drops of **Roman chamomile** to the *lavender* capsule if symptoms persist. During your hardest hit periods, take **Detoxification Blend** and **Digestive Enzyme Complex** daily as well.

DIFFUSE *lavender* at night and **Respiratory Blend** during the day to support restful breathing.

Essential oils are distilled versions of various plants, typically plants that are high in molecular compounds that are known to be beneficial to humans or animals. Distillation removes unwanted compounds (like allergens), and, ideally, what's left is all of the good and none of the bad components. Of course, that's only if the essential oil is a high quality, pure, therapeutic-grade oil. All essential oils are also gluten free.

Your Inner Geek

A study conducted in 2004 by the Department of Organic and Bio-organic Chemistry at Lund University in Sweden "showed the effectiveness of a nasal spray formulated with the essential oils of *eucalyptus* (cineole), *lavender* (linalool), and *cypress* (davanone) on upper airway disorders. After administration of the nasal spray, all patients experienced a rapid and significant relief of nasal symptoms, comparable to the effect of an antihistamine. Symptom relief was felt within 5 minutes after the administration of the spray and lasted for several hours."

> **If you are allergic to a thing, it is best not to put that thing in your mouth, particularly if the thing is cats. —Lemony Snicket**

Integrate

If your allergies are seasonal, start using the products listed in the 90-Day Plan Cheat Sheet one month before the season begins. Providing your body with essential oil–based nutritional supplements during that time may be just what you need to stay symptom free. Continue following the 90-Day Plan Cheat Sheet throughout the season. Maybe next year you can use less or even find that your allergies have disappeared!

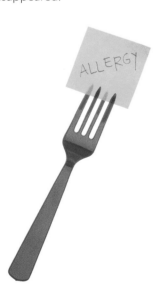

Did you know?

According to *National Geographic*, sneezes blast out germs and other unwanted intruders, but they also have another, just discovered purpose. A new study says when we breathe in foreign particles, sensors in our noses and sinuses detect the objects. The sensors signal the cilia—tiny hairlike paddles that line our nostrils and sinuses—to move to expel the irritants. This process is "always idling at first gear," with the cilia ready to spring into action when needed.

The study found that the burst of air produced by a sneeze not only clears nasal passages but also triggers the cilia sensors to kick the paddles into high gear for an extended period—about a couple of minutes. In that sense, a sneeze works by "resetting the system"—like an "escape" button on a computer.

≋ Dive In!

Wheat Belly: Lose the Wheat, Lose the Weight, and Find Your Path Back to Health by William Davis (Hardcover, 2011).

"The Allergy Buster: Can a Radical New Treatment Save Children With Severe Food Allergies?" by Melanie Thernstrom, *The New York Times,* March 7, 2013, Discussing a new treatment by Dr. Kari Nadeau, who is conducting a trial to desensitize children with multiple food allergies.

Cheat Sheet

MONTH 1
Respiratory Blend
Daily Supplements Pack
Detoxification Blend
Digestive Enzyme
Complex

MONTH 2
eucalyptus
lavender
Daily Supplements Pack
Digestive Enzyme
Complex

MONTH 3
Roman chamomile
lavender
Daily Supplements Pack
Digestive Enzyme
Complex

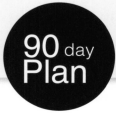

90 day **Plan**

Alzheimer's & Dementia

Alzheimer's disease is the most common form of dementia, a general term for loss of memory and other cognitive abilities serious enough to interfere with daily life. Alzheimer's accounts for 50 to 80 percent of all dementia cases. Parkinson's disease and other issues that affect the central nervous system are also often classified as dementia.

Our Approach

APPLY *frankincense* or *melissa* neat (undiluted) to the back of the neck frequently throughout the day. Apply **Focus Blend** on the temples and soles of the feet every morning.

TRY *Daily Supplements Pack* and **Essential Oil Cellular Complex** for nutritional support.

DIFFUSE *frankincense* at night and **Calming Blend** during the day to promote relaxation.

If your loved one suffers from irritability, try applying calming oils to the temples or feet while they are sleeping to improve their waking mood. Calming oils can also help caregivers cope with feelings of stress.

Your Inner Geek

"[As part of a] trial, lavender, geranium, and mandarin essential oils in an almond oil base were applied to the skin of 39 patients over an unspecified period. This resulted in increased alertness, contentment, and sleeping at night; and reduced levels of agitation, withdrawal, and wandering."
Journal of Advanced Nursing, 1995.

"In a recent, open-labelled trial on people with dementia, the use of a range of essential oils including ylang ylang, patchouli, rosemary, peppermint, and others produced a marked decrease in disturbed behavior in the majority of participants. This led to a reduction in prescribed conventional medicines, thereby delivering cost savings."
International Journal of Nursing Practice, 1998.

> ## Thou dewy dawn of memory.
> ### —Alfred Lord Tennyson

Integrate

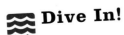 Depression and anxiety can affect those suffering from Alzheimer's and dementia, as well as their friends and families. Being on a wellness program that supports a positive mood can help you and your loved one deal better with the challenges you face.

The 90-Day Plan Cheat Sheet incorporates both a nutritional program and an oils program that can be used together or separately to lift the spirit!

Did you know?

The Alzheimer's Society reported the following in their *Journal of Quality Research in Dementia*:

- *Melissa* and lavender increased functional abilities and communication and decreased difficult behavior.
- *Lavender* aromatherapy with massage reduced frequency of excessive motor behavior.
- *Lavender* given to patients and placebo (water) on alternate days for ten days showed that the aromatherapy significantly reduced agitated behavior versus placebo.
- *Melissa* applied to the face and arms of patients, whilst other patients had sunflower oil applied, showed that *melissa* was associated with highly significant reductions in social withdrawal, together with an increase in constructive activities.
- *Lavender*, marjoram, patchouli, and vetiver applied as a cream to the body and limbs of patients compared with inert oil showed that the essential oil combination significantly increased alertness.

What is remarkable is that all essential oil treatments resulted in significant benefit, including (in most instances) reductions in agitation, sleeplessness, wandering, and unsociable behavior.

≈ Dive In!

Remember When? by Scientific American Editors (E-book, 2013).

"Could Hearing Loss and Dementia Be Connected?" by Pam Belluck, *The New York Times*, February 11, 2013.

Cheat Sheet

MONTH 1
frankincense
Daily Supplements Pack

MONTH 2
Focus Blend
Daily Supplements Pack

MONTH 3
melissa
Daily Supplements Pack
Calming Blend

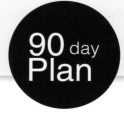

90 day **Plan**

Asthma

Asthma is a chronic inflammatory lung disease involving recurrent breathing problems. It affects more than 17 million people in the United States, and a third of these are children. Asthma affects people of all races and is slightly more common in African Americans, according to the National Institute of Allergy and Infectious Disease

Our Approach

APPLY *eucalyptus* or *Respiratory Blend* liberally to the chest, back, and bottoms of the feet morning and night (dilute for sensitive skin).

TRY the *Daily Supplements Pack* and *frankincense* and *lemon* oil (2 drops of each oil in a capsule, taken 2–4 times daily) to support the respiratory system.

DIFFUSE *Respiratory Blend* and *eucalyptus*, 15 minutes per day, to promote proper respiration. If you are extremely sensitive to scents, test a small amount of oil before you begin diffusing to see how you react. You can also apply the oil to the bottoms of your feet instead of diffusing. If you are experiencing an asthma attack, seek immediate attention from a medical professional.

Part of lessening an asthma attack is being able to stay calm. Incorporating deep breathing exercises not only strengthens the lungs but also calms the spirit.

Your Inner Geek

Professor Dr. Oliver Werz, Chair of Pharmaceutical and Medical Chemistry of the Friedrich Schiller University of Jena, Germany, is convinced that "the resin from the trunk of [frankincense] trees contains anti-inflammatory substances... These substances can be very beneficial in therapies against diseases like asthma, rheumatoid arthritis, or atopic dermatitis."

The Cleveland Clinic's website highlights a September 2009 study in *Phytotherapy Research*, which states, "Inflammation can be the underlying root of asthma and several other diseases including arthritis, gout, high blood pressure, kidney failure, colitis, and myocarditis. *Frankincense* can play an important role in relieving inflammation."

Integrate

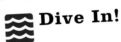 We recommend adding the products in the 90-Day Plan Cheat Sheet for Allergies if you have a severe case of asthma. Allergies and asthma are related, and you may find relief sooner using both. In addition, substitute natural cleaning products from our Cleaning section for the toxic chemicals found in most commercial cleaners. This can help to reduce potential asthma triggers in your home.

Did you know?

Asthma can be scary. Not knowing when an attack will strike can put the asthma sufferer in a constant state of concern, even panic. Stress can bring on an asthma attack and increase it once it has started. Try using a relaxing essential oil such as **lavender**. Carry **Calming Blend** with you during the day, and apply **eucalyptus** to your feet nightly to help balance your stress and fortify your lungs against an asthma attack. Once asthma strikes, you may not be able to breathe in these oils, so be proactive by applying oils to the feet when your asthma is under control.

≋ Dive In!

"Really? Breathing Exercises Can Relieve Asthma" by Anahad O'Connor, *The New York Times*, November 26, 2012.

"Kids With Asthma Play Hard, Too. In a Shift in Advice, Doctors Tell Patients to Get as Much Exercise as Their Peers" by Shirley S. Wang, *The Wall Street Journal*, April 22, 2013.

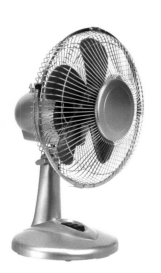

Cheat Sheet

MONTH 1
frankincense
lemon
Daily Supplements Pack

MONTH 2
eucalyptus
Calming Blend
Daily Supplements Pack

MONTH 3
Respiratory Blend
eucalyptus
Daily Supplements Pack

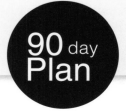

90 day
Plan

Autoimmune Disease Support

Autoimmune disease causes the body's protective force to attack itself. The name of the disease depends upon the location of the organ under attack. There are more than 100 known autoimmune diseases in the world today, and the list is growing.

Our Approach

APPLY *Soothing Rub* to help reduce body aches; apply *Protective Blend* (dilute for sensitive skin) to the bottoms of the feet to support immunity; and carry a *Soothing Blend* during the day to apply easily if pain strikes. Massage the spine daily with *Massage Blend*, neat (undiluted).

TRY 1 drop of *melissa* under the tongue 2–4 times a day. Take *Essential Oil Cellular Complex* once a day and the *Daily Supplements Pack* and *Digestive Enzyme Complex* capsule twice a day to help promote cellular health and balance nutrition.

DIFFUSE *Joyful Blend* during the day and *Calming Blend* at night to help you maintain a positive outlook.

Consider cleansing as part of your daily routine to help control inflammation. Taking *Essential Oil Omega Complex* or *Vegan Essential Oil Omega Complex* daily (part of the *Daily Supplements Pack* trio), which include a healthy amount of Omega-3, can help to reduce inflammation. For gentle daily cleansing, include *Digestive Enzyme Complex* between meals to help remove toxins.

Your Inner Geek

Need another reason to try *Essential Oil Cellular Complex,* which contains *lemongrass*? "*Lemongrass* is effective in treating various types of cancers without affecting the healthy normal cells of the body. Research conducted to prove the anti-cancer activity of lemongrass has shown promise in the prevention of skin cancer. Studies have also shown that the component citral, present in lemongrass, helps in inhibiting the growth of hepatic [liver] cancer cells during the initial phases and prevents any further production. Another study has provided supportive evidence regarding the anti-proliferative effect of citral in impeding the growth of human breast cancer cells and induction of apoptosis [cell death]." *OrganicFacts.net.*

> **Every human being is the author of his own health or disease.**
> **—Buddha**

Integrate

 Incorporating the supplement plan in the 90-Day Plan Cheat Sheet on Nutrition is an easy way to enrich the diet of anyone with an autoimmune disease. Better nutrition can also increase the length and quality of sleep, an important element of healing.

Did you know?

Bringing up your energy level can be almost as beneficial as putting the disease in remission. Taking **Cellular Vitality Complex** (part of the **Daily Supplements Pack**) may help support healthy cell proliferation and lifespan, mitochondrial energy production, and healthy cellular inflammatory response—helping to raise your energy level so that you can feel normal again.

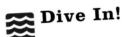 **Dive In!**

"Salt Intake Tied to Autoimmune Diseases," *The New York Times News Service*, March 7, 2013.

"The Boy With a Thorn in His Joints". by Susannah Meadows, *New York Times Magazine*, February 1, 2013.

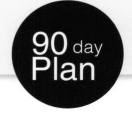

Cheat Sheet

MONTH 1
Essential Oil Cellular Complex
Soothing Rub
Daily Supplements Pack
Protective Blend
Digestive Enzyme Complex

MONTH 2
Essential Oil Cellular Complex
Joyful Blend
Daily Supplements Pack
melissa
Digestive Enzyme Complex

MONTH 3
Massage Blend
Essential Oil Cellular Complex
Soothing Roll-on
Daily Supplements Pack
Calming Blend
Digestive Enzyme Complex

90 day **Plan**

Blood Pressure

About one in three adults in the United States has high blood pressure (HBP). Often, without symptoms, a person can have HBP for years without knowing it. Over time, this "silent" condition can damage the heart, blood vessels, kidneys, and other parts of the body.

Our Approach

APPLY 1–2 drops of *cypress*, *helichrysum, ylang ylang*, and *Calming Blend*, neat (undiluted), over the heart.

TRY a *Trim Shake* as a meal substitute, which may help you to balance your blood pressure and reduce your salt intake.

DIFFUSE *ylang ylang*, *bergamot*, or *Calming Blend* to clear the mind and reduce pressure and stress.

Your Inner Geek

According to the *European Journal of Preventive Cardiology*, Taiwan, 2012, "The essential oils which form the basis of aromatherapy for stress relief are also reported to have a beneficial effect on heart rate and blood pressure following short-term exposure—and may, therefore, reduce the risk of cardiovascular disease."

In the book *Advanced Aromatherapy*, author Kurt Schnaubelt, PhD, notes that "even in the minutest amounts, ylang ylang has a marked and immediate effect on heart palpitations."

Including lots of fresh potassium-rich fruits and vegetables in your daily diet is an important part of any blood pressure—lowering program. Aim for potassium levels of up to 4,000 mg a day, says Linda Van Horn, PhD, RD, professor of preventive medicine at University Feinberg School of Medicine. Potassium rich foods include tomatoes, raisins, spinach, and beans.

A man goes to a doctor for a physical checkup. The nurse starts with certain basic items. "How much do you weigh?" she asks. "One-seventy." The nurse puts him on the scale. It turns out that his weight is 183. The nurse asks, "Your height?" "Five-eleven." The nurse checks and sees that he's only 5' 8 1/2". She then takes his blood pressure, and it's very high. The man explains, "Of course it's high. When I came in here, I was tall and wiry. Now, I'm short and dumpy."

Integrate

For extra support, try our easy nutritional program in the Weight Management section and follow the 90-Day Plan Cheat Sheet. Our program gives you a weight loss guide for foods, oils, and supplements that may help you achieve healthy blood pressure.

Did you know?

Dealing with stress is key to maintaining healthy blood pressure. If you struggle with stress, pick one task in your day that you can eliminate or share with someone who can help you. Trying to lose weight to decrease your blood pressure? Instead of sharing a meal with a friend, ask them to help you with a fun or small task around your house, go on an errand you have to run, or even take a walk together instead of sitting with a cup of coffee. This will give you some time with your friend while avoiding the high-fat/high-salt trap of restaurant food. Managing work and tasks with others reduces stress. Incorporate stress-reducing oils like *lavender*, *bergamot*, and *Calming Blend* to help your blood pressure stay in a healthy range.

 Dive In!

"High Blood Pressure Tied to Brain Changes" by Nicholas Bakalar, *The New York Times*, November 12, 2012.

The Blood Pressure Cure: 8 Weeks to Lower Blood Pressure without Prescription Drugs by Robert E. Kowalski (Paperback, 2008).

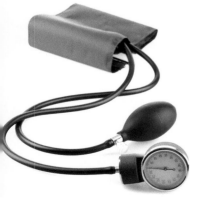

Cheat Sheet

MONTH 1
cypress
helichrysum
Trim Shake
ylang ylang

MONTH 2
bergamot
Trim Shake
ylang ylang

MONTH 3
cypress
Trim Shake
Calming Blend

90 day Plan

Brain Power

When you feel foggy, forgetful, or scattered, it may be time to feed your brain. The brain, made up mostly of fat, will perform at its highest level only when well fed. Our brain not only controls how we think but also how our body systems perform. Complex disorders in the central nervous system can lead to autism, ADD, ADHD, Alzheimer's disease, and other neurological issues.

Our Approach

APPLY *Focus Blend* to the soles of the feet, and apply *Grounding Blend* and *Calming Blend* or *frankincense* neat to the spine. Apply **helichrysum**, **sandalwood**, **vetiver**, **patchouli,** and **melissa** neat to the brain stem (at the nape of the neck) for additional support to the central nervous system. Carry *Focus Blend* with you, and apply it during the day for extra support.

TRY the *Daily Supplements Pack* and *Essential Oil Cellular Complex* 1–2 times daily. *Digestive Enzyme Complex* can help with digestion and nutrient assimilation to build a healthy body, which yields a healthy brain.

DIFFUSE *frankincense* day and night. You can also substitute *lavender* or *Calming Blend* to help you sleep more soundly.

Researchshows that students who study late at night on caffeine find their short-term memory fails them on the next day's exam (January 2009 issue of *Behavioral Sleep Medicine*). Skip the coffee, and pop a **Peppermint Beadlet** instead; or put a drop of **peppermint** on the tongue and another on the back of the neck. You can repeat this every 20 minutes until you feel revived.

Your Inner Geek

"Low levels of omega-3 fatty acids were… associated with poor test scores for visual memory, problem solving, multi-tasking, and abstract thinking. It is thought that omega-3 fatty acids in fish oils may reduce inflammation of the brain and play a part in brain development and nerve cell regeneration," notes Dr. Zaldy Tan, an Alzheimer's researcher from the University of California at Los Angeles, who led the US research reported in the journal *Neurology*. "People with lower blood levels of omega-3 fatty acids had lower brain volumes… equivalent to about two years of structural brain aging."

In studies conducted at Vienna and Berlin Universities, researchers found that "sesquiterpenes, a natural compound found in essential oils of vetiver, patchouli, sandalwood, and frankincense, can increase levels of oxygen in the brain by up to 28 percent" (Nasel, 1992). "Such an increase in brain oxygen may lead to a heightened level of activity in

Did you know?

Although the causes of ADD/ADHD are controversial, there is general agreement about what can help. Regular exercise, such as walking or riding a bike, and getting enough sleep are critical. Limiting electronics can also help ensure a healthy amount of sleep, as can calming oils like **Calming Blend** and **lavender**. Include a comprehensive dietary supplement for children that is rich in fish oil, like **Omega-3 Fish Oil**, and B vitamins, like **Chewable Multivitamins**. Another troubling ailment that affects the brain is Autism. Consider adding enzymes to the diet. Taken before meals, enzymes are effective at improving symptoms such as attention deficit, socialization, hyperactivity, eye contact, comprehension, and compulsions (Timothy Buie, MD, Pediatric Gastroenterology, Harvard/Mass General Hospital).

Andrew Weil, MD, recommends making sure that children with autism get sufficient omega-3 fatty acids. Recent research indicates that supplementing the diet with these beneficial fats can help address autism as well as depression, bipolar disorder, and attention deficit hyperactivity disorder.

the hypothalamus and limbic systems of the brain, which can have dramatic effects on not only emotions but on learning, attitude, and many physical processes of the body, such as immune function, hormone balance, and energy levels. High levels of sesquiterpenes also occur in *melissa*, *myrrh*, and *clove* essential oils."

Integrate

Take a look at the section on Cleaning to learn how to replace dangerous chemical cleaners and personal care products, which may exacerbate neurological issues, with natural alternatives—healthy home, healthy mind. Children with autism can also benefit from probiotics, which contain the helpful bacteria that normally inhabit the human digestive tract. Probiotics can decrease leakage of large molecules from the gut that can trigger immune reactions with effects on brain function.

Dive In!

Luminosity.com or *Mental Floss Magazine*.

The A.D.D. Book: New Understandings, New Approaches to Parenting Your Child by William Sears and Lynda Thompson (Paperback, 1998).

Mental Floss Presents: Condensed Knowledge: A Deliciously Irreverent Guide to Feeling Smart Again" by Will Pearson, Mangesh Hattikudur, and Elizabeth Hunt (Paperback, 2004).

Cheat Sheet

MONTH 1
Grounding Blend
Essential Oil Cellular Complex
Focus Blend
Daily Supplements Pack
melissa
Digestive Enzyme Complex

MONTH 2
frankincense
Essential Oil Cellular Complex
Daily Supplements Pack
Calming Blend
Digestive Enzyme Complex
vetiver

MONTH 3
Essential Oil Cellular Complex
helichrysum
Daily Supplements Pack
patchouli
sandalwood
Digestive Enzyme Complex

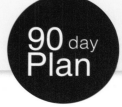

90 day **Plan**

Breast Health

Know your breasts. Changes in breast shape, size, and feel are common, and many changes are benign. Conduct regular breast self-examinations, and stay in close contact with your doctor about your breast health so you can detect any problem early.

Our Approach

APPLY 1 drop each of *frankincense*, *lavender*, *rosemary,* and *sandalwood* neat, daily, to each breast for breast health support. If you are experiencing a hormone imbalance, apply **Women's Monthly Blend** to abdomen, chest, or back of neck throughout the day for symptoms associated with PMS or menopause.

TRY the **Daily Supplements Pack** capsules to maintain proper nutrition. Take 1–2 drops of **orange** in water daily to help fight free radical damage. Add **Essential Oil Cellular Complex** to your daily routine if you have a history of breast health concerns.

DIFFUSE *lavender* at night to promote good sleep and healthy cell regeneration.

Any meal or snack high in carbohydrates generates a rapid rise in blood glucose. Cancers feed on sugar. Limiting your intake of sugars can help reduce your cancer risk. Be mindful of meals or snacks high in fructose (from fruit), lactose (from milk or soft cheese), or starchy carbohydrates (bread, pasta), which can generate a rapid rise in blood glucose. Just remember the rule for cheese: the harder the cheese, the less moisture and whey it contains, thus less lactose. Hard cheese has not only been drained of its whey/lactose, but much of that is converted to lactic acid during the beginning of the cheese-making process, thereby reducing the amount of lactose (sugar) present. Taking Digestive Enzyme Complex capsules daily with meals may help you process the sugars you eat more effectively.

Your Inner Geek

Several studies have been conducted to establish a link between **rosemary** and breast cancer prevention. "Crude…extracts of rosemary have the ability to prevent the proliferation of breast cancer cells in the laboratory," report the researchers in the journal *Oncology Reports*, June 2007. In addition, the B*razilian Journal of Microbiology*, October–December 2010, notes that "along with the anti-proliferative activity, rosemary essential oil contains significant antioxidant properties to stabilize free radicals. This is important, as unstable free radicals may interact with the components of healthy cells and turn them into cancerous ones."

Randy Jirlte, PhD, Duke University Medical Center Radiology Oncology, cites from "Regression of Mammalian Carcinomas" by Gould and Crowell, "High doses of d-limonene [found in citrus oils] increase the production and activation of [the] protein TGF-beta that actually program[s] breast cancer cells to self destruct."

Integrate

Are household cleaners linked to breast cancer? In a study published recently in the Journal of Environmental Health, breast cancer risk was highest among women who reported the greatest use of cleaning products and air fresheners. The risk was twice that of those who reported low use of these products. Replace candles and chemical air fresheners with a diffuser filled with your favorite essential oil or blend, and use the products suggested in the Cleaning section to get started!

Did you know?

You can make a date with yourself for breast health! Every October (during Breast Cancer Awareness Month) and April (6 months later), follow the 90-Day Plan Cheat Sheet for Breast Health. Apply *frankincense*, *lavender*, *rosemary,* and *sandalwood* neat to the breasts every day for the entire month (approximately one drop per breast each day; dilute with *coconut oil* if you experience any discomfort). Use up all 4 essential oils by the end of the month. Be generous: this is the best gift you can give yourself, a friend, or sister! In addition, take *orange* essential oil in capsules during the month, also using up the bottle (about 5–6 drops per day).

≈ Dive In!

Dr. Susan Love's Breast Book, 5th Edition by Susan M. Love, MD, and Karen Lindsey (Paperback, 2010).

Mother-Daughter Wisdom: Understanding the Crucial Link Between Mothers, Daughters, and Health by Christiane Northrup, MD (Paperback, 2006).

Cheat Sheet

MONTH 1
Essential Oil Cellular Complex
coconut oil
frankincense
lavender
Daily Supplements Pack
sandalwood

MONTH 2
Essential Oil Cellular Complex
Daily Supplements Pack
rosemary
orange

MONTH 3
Essential Oil Cellular Complex
lavender
Daily Supplements Pack
Women's Monthly Blend

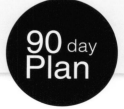

90 day **Plan**

Bug Bites & Repellents

Bugs can transmit diseases to you and your pets. Although not every bite is toxic, it is certainly best to avoid them, as they are generally uncomfortable. If you are bitten, be sure to find out what bit you and, if necessary, have it tested.

Our Approach

APPLY *Repellent Blend* to exposed skin and openings in clothing before outdoor activity. If bitten or stung, apply *Cleansing Blend* around the bite to reduce swelling and draw out any infection or toxins. Apply *Soothing Blend* around the bite to reduce pain and inflammation. Apply *Protective Blend* to the bottoms of your feet twice a day, and repeat as needed.

TRY taking *GI Cleansing Formula* after being bitten. If the bite or sting has not healed, continue immune support by taking a *Probiotic Defense Formula* capsule. Get in the habit of taking the *Daily Supplements Pack* to build the body's fortification against toxins and infections.

DIFFUSE by placing cotton balls with 5–10 drops of *peppermint* on them by doors, attics, foundation cracks, and windows (change every 2–4 weeks). This may help keep spiders, ants, and other insects from entering your home. *Repellent Blend* also helps to keep bugs from coming back. Put 5–10 drops of *Repellent Blend* on cotton balls, and strategically place them around your picnic table, patio, or outdoor activity area to keep away pests. This is a must-have for campers and outdoor athletes!

Your Inner Geek

A study by University of Cartagena, Colombia, found, "The use of synthetic chemicals to control insects and arthropods raises several concerns related to environment and human health.

"In contrast, essential oils from plants belonging to several species have been extensively tested to assess their repellent properties as a valuable natural resource." Individual compounds (like the ones found in *Repellent Blend*) show "high repellent activity, including alpha-pinene, limonene, citronellol, citronellal, camphor, and thymol."

"Plant-based repellents have been used for generations in traditional practice as a personal protection measure against host-seeking mosquitoes. Recently, commercial repellent products containing plant-based ingredients have gained increasing popularity among consumers." Apply frequently for best results.
Malaria Journal, 2011

> To make a prairie it takes a clover and one bee, One clover, and a bee,
> and revery. The revery alone will do, if bees are few.
> —Emily Dickinson

Integrate

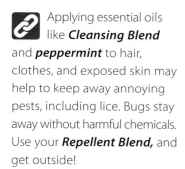 Applying essential oils like **Cleansing Blend** and **peppermint** to hair, clothes, and exposed skin may help to keep away annoying pests, including lice. Bugs stay away without harmful chemicals. Use your **Repellent Blend,** and get outside!

To repel pests, apply an essential oil such as **Repellent Blend** (or other type of conifer oil, like **spruce** or **white fir**). Give special attention to the warmest, leanest parts of the body: neck, armpits, ears, wrists, or wherever blood vessels are close to the surface.

Did you know?

We have traveled all over the world; and no matter where we go, there are always bugs. Eating the foods of the region and avoiding sugars is one way to keep bugs at bay. You want to smell like a local!

Taking oils internally that repel bugs, like **peppermint**, can also help keep pests away as the oils begin to perspire from your pores. If you are bitten or stung, put a drop of **Calming Blend** around the bite.

For ticks, apply a drop of **oregano** over the bite, and wait a minute until the tick releases. Pick up the tick quickly with a clean tissue, and dispose of it properly—in a toilet or boiling water! Apply **melaleuca** at the site of the bite, and cover the area with a small bandage. Observe the area daily, and see a physician if a rash develops or other symptoms appear. The oils in **Calming Blend**, including **lavender** and **Roman chamomile**, act as an antihistamine and may help to prevent an allergic reaction.

Don't just apply your oils once. Swimming and perspiring will diminish the effect of any oil. Apply your oils often to provide the protection you need.

≋ Dive In!

"Bugged Out" by Bonnie Rochman, *Time Magazine*, Sunday March 27, 2011.

"How a Leafy Folk Remedy Stopped Bedbugs in Their Tracks" by Felicity Barringer, *New York Times*, April 9, 2013.

Cheat Sheet

MONTH 1
Soothing Blend
Daily Supplements Pack
peppermint
Cleansing Blend
Repellent Blend

MONTH 2
Protective Blend
Daily Supplements Pack
Repellent Blend

MONTH 3
GI Cleansing Formula
Daily Supplements Pack
Probiotic Defense Formula
Cleansing Blend
Repellent Blend

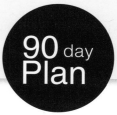

90 day **Plan**

Burns

There are 3 types of burns: first, second, and third degree burns. The first degree burn does not burn through the outer layer of skin, the second degree burns through only the first layer, and the third degree burns through all layers: skin, fat, and even, at times, bone. Be sure to know the type of burn you have. Burns should receive a proper diagnosis and immediate medical attention.

Our Approach

APPLY *lavender* and *melaleuca* around, never on, the affected area. To help with the pain, apply a **Soothing Blend** and *cypress* on the soles of the feet (not near the wound). Once the wound scabs over, apply *frankincense*, *helichrysum*, or *lavender,* and top with a little bit of **lip balm** to create a moisture seal.

TRY the **Daily Supplements Pack** 2 times a day. Take 2 drops each of *clove*, *helichrysum*, *vetiver*, and *frankincense* in a capsule to help minimize the pain.

DIFFUSE *lavender* or a **Grounding Blend** to reduce stress.

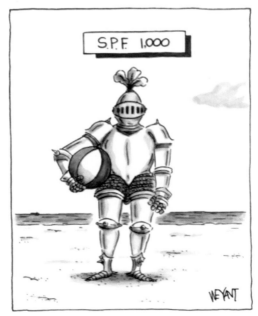

Your Inner Geek

According to the University of Maryland Medical Center, "People who get burned are very prone to infection. It can be hard to tell if a minor burn is infected because the skin surrounding a burn is usually red and may become warm to the touch—both of which are also signs of infection. Any change in the appearance of a burn, or in the way that the person feels, should be brought to the attention of a doctor. Potential signs of infection include: change in color of the burnt area or surrounding skin; purplish discoloration, particularly if swelling is also present; change in thickness of the burn (the burn suddenly extends deep into the skin); greenish discharge, pus, or fever."

> **The mind is not a vessel to be filled but a fire to be kindled**
> **—Plutarch**

Integrate

Burns must be well tended to heal. Taking care of the skin—keeping it clean, protected, and free from infection—is key. We like to keep **melaleuca** around for burns. Whether your burn is from the sun or from the stove, **melaleuca** on the soles of your feet and around the burn will help to keep infection away. Have your oils on hand to be prepared in case of an emergency.

Mild sunburns can be soothed with a homemade blend of a natural aloe vera gel (available at most health food stores) mixed with a drop of **lavender** essential oil, both known skin-healing agents. Wearing light-colored clothing and a hat that covers your skin is the best protection from the sun. Sunscreen should be used sparingly—look for a natural option if possible. Foods with beta carotene, such as carrots and squash, help to build natural sun protection in the skin.

Did you know?

When choosing a sunscreen, do you know what to look for? Over $800 million is spent annually in the United States on sunscreen; and while there are over 1,800 products on the market, many offer poor protection from sun damage and often contain toxic ingredients. The Environmental Working Group in their annual review of sunscreens offers the following advice: look for a product containing zinc oxide with an SPF 15 to 50, depending on your skin tone and sun intensity. Use lotions, not sprays or powders, for greatest effectiveness. Avoid sunscreens containing Vitamin A, which has been shown to cause skin cancer in laboratory tests, or oxybenzone, a hormone disrupter and skin allergen. Last but not least, products with an SPF higher than 50 offer little additional benefit.

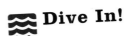 **Dive In!**

"The Sun's Unrelenting Rays, Do Animals Get Sunburned?" by C. Claiborne Ray, *The New York Times*, May 14, 2012.

"How Tanning Changes the Brain" by Anahad O'Connor, *The New York Times*, April 12, 2011.

Cheat Sheet

MONTH 1
Soothing Blend
lavender
Daily Supplements Pack
melaleuca

MONTH 2
cypress
frankincense
Daily Supplements Pack
Calming Blend

MONTH 3
clove
helichrysum
lip balm
Daily Supplements Pack
vetiver

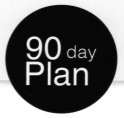

90 day **Plan**

Don't forget the old adage: The best defense is a good offense. Cancer takes on many different forms and displays various symptoms. The recommendations here are for general health support and to strengthen the body's defenses for those who want to prevent, are addressing, or are recovering from cancer. As always, all natural products should be used under the advisement of your health care professional.

Our Approach

APPLY 4 drops of any of the following oils: *frankincense*, *orange*, *lavender*, *thyme*, *myrrh*, *lemongrass*, *sandalwood*, *rosemary*, *clove* and/or *Essential Oil Cellular Complex* to your feet or along the spine. Dilute if the skin is sensitive.

TRY the *Daily Supplements Pack* and *Digestive Enzyme Complex* before each meal, and take a 1/2 capsule of *orange* 2 times daily.

DIFFUSE *lavender* or *Grounding Blend* to reduce stress.

Ginger root contains compounds that may help relieve or prevent nausea and vomiting. These substances can increase the flow of saliva and digestive juices. They may also help to calm the stomach and intestines after treatments.

Your Inner Geek

Exciting research is being done on essential oil antitumor properties and their specific anticancer action. A search of PubMed, the National Institute of Health's online research database, produces 498 results for the search "essential oils cancer" and 572 results for "essential oils tumor." Many of the studies show a direct correlation of tumor and cancer cell line eradication and have conclusions that indicate the need for further investigation into the development of accepted therapies using essential oils.

According to the American Cancer Society, "Clinical studies suggest aromatherapy may be a helpful complementary therapy. In Britain, there are reports of the successful use of aromatherapy massage in people who have cancer to reduce anxiety, depression, tension, and pain. There are also reports that breathing the

> **The body is like a piano, and happiness is like music. It is needful to have the instrument in good order. —Henry Ward Beecher**

vapors of peppermint, ginger, and cardamom oil seems to relieve the nausea caused by chemotherapy and radiation."

Integrate

A 2009 Stanford University School of Medicine study found a link between cancer recurrence and early death in patients who also suffer from depression. Fortify your health with products to support your mood. The 90-Day Plan Cheat Sheet for Depression will give you a program of oils and supplements to keep your spirits high during times of struggle and challenge. This program is also helpful for caretakers and family members.

Did you know?

Here are some additional products you may want to add to your regimen for symptom relief:

- Anxiety: *Grounding Blend*, *Calming Blend,* and *Joyful Blend* (on the pulse points)
- Dry Skin: *Hand and Body Lotion* mixed with *lavender* and *geranium* (for the whole body)
- Exhaustion: *Tension Blend* (on the nape of the neck)
- Hair Loss: *Protecting Shampoo* and *Smoothing Conditioner* (for safe, gentle cleaning)
- Insomnia: *Calming Blend* (on the nape of the neck)
- Mouth sores: *Protective Toothpaste* (for gentle non-toxic cleaning)
- Nausea: *ginger* or *peppermint* (a drop on the tongue, or diffuse)
- Pain: *Soothing Blend* or *Soothing Rub* (at the site of pain or around if there is a wound)

90 day **Plan**

Dive In!

"Our Feel-Good War on Breast Cancer" by Peggy Orenstein, *The New York Times*, April 25, 2013.

"Using Data to Treat Cancer and Drive Innovation: How a Pair of Savvy Renegades Are Forcing Collaboration in Cancer R&D and Saving Lives" Creative Conversations by Linda Tischler, *Fast Company*, April 15, 2013.

Cheat Sheet

MONTH 1
Grounding Blend
Essential Oil Cellular Complex
Soothing Blend
ginger
peppermint
rosemary
Daily Supplements Pack
thyme
orange

MONTH 2
clove
Essential Oil Cellular Complex
frankincense
geranium
Hand & Body Lotion
lavender
Daily Supplements Pack
myrrh
Calming Blend

MONTH 3
Essential Oil Cellular Complex
lemongrass
Daily Supplements Pack
Protective Toothpaste
Tension Blend
Protecting Shampoo
Smoothing Conditioner
sandalwood
orange

Candida & Yeast Infection

Candida and yeast are microorganisms that live in every human body. Problems arise when yeast becomes unbalanced. Many factors can contribute to this, including medications, diet, genetics, age, hydration, and more. Finding a solution is individual, but the suggestions here may support you on your path to wellness.

Our Approach

APPLY *Melaleuca alternifolia* and **oregano** diluted to the bottoms of the feet. **Oregano** is an excellent oil for children, too. Of course, always dilute oils for children. If you can keep your kids out of the current trend of over-prescribed antibiotics and heavy sugar consumption, you will go a long way to avoiding yeast overgrowth in their bodies. Bathe with a *Invigorating Bath Bar*.

TRY 3 drops of **cassia** under the tongue before meals and 1 drop of **clove** on the tip of the tongue to reduce sugar cravings. Try *GI Cleansing Formula* and *Detoxification Blend* along with the *Daily Supplements Pack* and *Probiotic Defense Formula* daily to help create an environment unfavorable for yeast. Also, try *Digestive Enzyme Complex* capsules with every meal to promote healthy digestion.

DIFFUSE *peppermint* to reduce cravings caused by yeast overgrowth

Mom & Baby Note: Thrush usually develops suddenly, but it may become chronic, persisting over a long period of time. A common sign of thrush is the presence of creamy white, slightly raised lesions in the mouth—usually on the tongue or inner cheeks.

Your Inner Geek

"A test tube study demonstrated that oregano oil and an extract in the oil called carvacrol, in particular, inhibited the growth of *Candida albicans* far more effectively than a commonly employed antifungal agent called calcium magnesium caprylate." *University of Michigan Health System.*

"In other words, probiotic bacteria [like those in *Probiotic Defense Formula*] are effective in controlling Candida in the mouth, a problem of particular concern for the elderly. The exact mechanism by which probiotics inhibit Candida growth is not fully understood to date. Some suggest the ability of probiotics to produce hydrogen peroxide plays a role; however, in vivo studies suggest that probiotics might prevent Candida growth through multiple mechanisms." *Probiotic Rescue: How You can use Probiotics to Fight Cholesterol,*

> **Coconut oil is truly the healthiest oil you can consume. It is rich in lauric acid, which is known for being antiviral, antibacterial, and antifungal.**
> —Dr. Joseph Mercola, MD

Cancer, Superbugs, Digestive Complaints and More by Allison Tannis (Paperback, 2008).

Integrate

Eat an alkaline diet. Alkaline foods include fresh fruits and vegetables, sea salt, and molasses. Adding probiotics to your diet can also help keep Candida at bay. Follow our easy program in the 90-Day Plan Cheat Sheet in the section on Weight Management. Our program gives yeast a run for its money. Eating the right foods keeps your body balanced, which is the key to managing naturally-occurring yeast.

Drugs that can wipe out intestinal flora or encourage overgrowth of yeast include steroids and estrogen, either in the form of birth control pills or hormone replacement therapy. Andrew Weil, MD

Did you know?

Candida albicans is a yeast that occurs naturally in the body. The body's natural defenses normally keep yeast in check; but if there is an imbalance, the yeast can grow out of control. Candida thrives in warm moist places such as the mouth, vagina, or between folds of the skin. Cleansing the skin with **Invigorating Bath Bar** can keep Candida off the skin. Using a topical soap as well as nutritional supplements and an essential oil program can help to balance your body, both inside and out. According to the University of Maryland, about 75 percent of women will get a vaginal yeast infection in their lifetime.

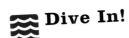 **Dive In!**

Eight Weeks to Optimum Health: A Proven Program for Taking Full Advantage of Your Body's Natural Healing Power by Andrew Weil MD (Paperback 2007).

The Fungus Link by Doug Kaufman (Paperback, 2008).

Cheat Sheet

MONTH 1
coconut oil
GI Cleansing Formula
Daily Supplements Pack
melaleuca
oregano
Probiotic Defense Formula
Digestive Enzyme Complex

MONTH 2
cassia
Invigorating Bath Bar
clove
Probiotic Defense Formula
Digestive Enzyme Complex
Daily Supplements Pack
Detoxification Blend

MONTH 3
Probiotic Defense Formula
peppermint
Daily Supplements Pack
Digestive Enzyme Complex

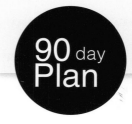

90 day Plan

Cholesterol

If we are all different, then it stands to reason that we should all have different cholesterol levels. However, standard practice today says everyone should have the same number. In addition, cholesterol at the right level can play a positive role in the body. Keeping your cholesterol at a healthy level can be supported with oils and nutrition.

Our Approach

APPLY 1–2 drops of **cypress, helichrysum,** and **ylang ylang** neat over the heart and on the bottoms of the feet. Apply **Massage Blend** neat to the back of the neck daily.

TRY the **Daily Supplements Pack** and **Digestive Enzyme Complex** capsules daily. Try 1–4 drops of **Metabolic Blend**, in capsules, daily to help burn unwanted fat.

DIFFUSE *lavender* to promote a full night's sleep so that the body can regulate its own cholesterol.

The *Harvard Medical School Guide to Healthy Eating* suggests that consuming cinnamon essential oil (*Cinnamomum cassia*) could reduce your cholesterol by 12 to 30 percent.

Your Inner Geek

According to Ronald Ross Watson, author of the book *Vegetables, Fruits, and Herbs in Health Promotion,* "Essential oils that contain terpenoid compounds such as geraniol and citral decrease cholesterol levels. These compounds inhibit the production of mevalonic acid, an intermediary in the production of cholesterol and the target of many cholesterol-lowering pharmaceutical drugs.

"In addition, getting at least 8 hours of sleep is essential to lower your cholesterol and heart disease risk. A good night's sleep helps to heal your body, maintains the blood sugar level and improves your overall health and mental health." *Times of India*, March 2013.

"Common and cassia cinnamon have both been reported to have anti-diabetic and lipid-lowering effects. The objective was to determine if the combination of common and cassia cinnamon reduces

Did you know?

The link between *lemongrass* essential oil and cholesterol was investigated by researchers from the Department of Nutritional Sciences, University of Wisconsin. They published their findings in the medical journal, *Lipids*. In the 90-day study, one group characterized as the responders experienced on average a 25 point drop in cholesterol after one month, which continued over the course of the study. After 3 months, cholesterol levels among the responders had decreased by a significant 38 points. Once the responders stopped taking the *lemongrass,* their cholesterol returned to previous levels.

fasting blood glucose, insulin, glycosylated hemoglobin (HA1C), triglyceride, total cholesterol, HDL cholesterol and LDL cholesterol levels in people with type 2 diabetes." *BMC Complementary and Alternative Medicine*, 2012.

Integrate

Essential oils are incredible multi-taskers. Taking an oil for one issue often improves another. We recommend using our fat burning oils to lose weight and reduce your cholesterol. Try our easy program in the 90-Day Plan Cheat Sheet in the section on Weight Management. Our program gives you a fat burning guide for foods, oils, and supplements.

Dive In!

The Great Cholesterol Myth: Why Lowering Your Cholesterol Won't Prevent Heart Disease-and the Statin-Free Plan That Will by Jonny Bowden and Stephen Sinatra (Paperback, 2012).

"Not So Young at Heart" by Ron Wilson, *Wall Street Journal*, August 3, 2010.

Cheat Sheet

MONTH 1
Massage Blend
Daily Supplements Pack
Metabolic Blend
Digestive Enzyme
Complex

MONTH 2
cypress
helichrysum
Daily Supplements Pack
Metabolic Blend
Digestive Enzyme
Complex

MONTH 3
Daily Supplements Pack
Metabolic Blend
Digestive Enzyme
Complex
ylang ylang

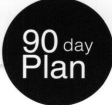

90 day **Plan**

Cleaning

Essential oils have been used for cleaning for centuries. Their antipathogenic properties keep your home, vehicle, and workplace clean and smelling fresh.

Our Approach

APPLY diluted *Protective Cleaner* to any surface. Always spot test first. For mold or for tough stains, use a 50/50 dilution with water. For glass cleaning, add a cup of vinegar and one capful of *Protective Cleaner* to a 32 oz. spray bottle filled with water. We love using *Protective Hand Wash* for bathrooms, classrooms, kitchens, and more!

Use *Protective Laundry Detergent* to reduce your exposure to potential allergens and toxins in your home or on clothes and skin. For an added benefit, use a washcloth with a drop or two of your favorite essential oil instead of chemically laden dryer sheets. We like to use *Protective Blend* to help keep germs and odors off of towels and sports clothes and *lavender* or *orange* for linens and sleepwear.

TRY the *Daily Supplements Pack* and *Digestive Enzyme Complex* before each meal, and take a 1/2 capsule of *orange* 2 times daily.

DIFFUSE *lavender* or *Grounding Blend* to reduce stress.

Melaleuca and *grapefruit* are great oils to add to your *Protective Cleaner* solution or bucket of soapy water. You can add these germ killers to sponges, dishwater, and the clothes dryer. This is especially good to do when you have a sick person at home.

Your Inner Geek

"Out of 21 essential oils tested, 19 oils showed antibacterial activity against one or more strains. *Cinnamon*, *clove*, *geranium*, *lemon*, *lime*, *orange,* and *rosemary* oils exhibited significant inhibitory effects. *Cinnamon* oil showed promising inhibitory activity even at low concentration." *BMC Complementary and Alternative Medicine*, 2006.

"Essential oils (EOs) have been long recognized for their antibacterial, antifungal, antiviral, insecticidal, and antioxidant properties. EOs and their components show promising activities against many food-borne pathogens and spoilage microorganisms when tested in vitro." *Molecules*, Université de Ouagadougou, Burkina Faso, 2012.

Integrate

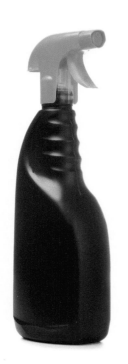

Greening your home with natural cleaning products is a great way to start improving your health! Visit our social media sites often to see recipes for cleaning every room in your home.

Did you know?

Cleaning with different commercial cleaners can pose a great risk to your health. Chemicals can linger in the air for up to two weeks and, when combined with other cleaners, can cause a toxic cloud in your home. Residues from cleaners also leave behind dangerous toxins that your children, pets, family, and friends can inhale. Beware of synthetic air fresheners, scented candles, and dryer sheets: they can be just as toxic as the odors they attempt to mask. In contrast, **Protective Cleaner** is safe on most surfaces and will not leave a toxic residue. Watch out for laundry detergents that have petroleum distillates or napthas. These chemicals have been linked to cancer, lung damage, and/or inflammation, and mucous membrane damage. Choose **Protective Laundy Detergent** instead.

≋ Dive In!

Gorgeously Green: 8 Simple Steps to an Earth Friendly Life by Sophie Uliano (Paperback, 2008).

Green This! Volume 1: Greening Your Cleaning by Deidre Imus (Paperback, 2007).

Cheat Sheet

MONTH 1
lemon
Cleansing Blend
Protective Toothpaste
Protective Hand Wash
Protective Cleaner

MONTH 2
Invigorating Blend
Protective Toothpaste
Protective Hand Wash
Protective Laundry Detergent

MONTH 3
grapefruit
Protective Toothpaste
Protective Hand Wash
Protective Cleaner

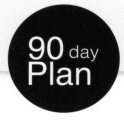

90 day Plan

Colds

Colds contribute to more lost work and school days than any other illness. Typically lasting 21 days, and caused by viruses, a cold can linger, depressing the spirits as well as the body. Get to it fast, and stop it in its tracks.

Our Approach

APPLY *Protective Blend*, *Cleansing Blend*, and *Detoxification Blend* to the feet in rotating order. Apply **eucalyptus** or **Respiratory Blend** to the chest and back. Wipe off household surfaces, including telephones, light switches, and doorknobs with diluted **Protective Cleaner**.

TRY the *Daily Supplements Pack* and **Protective Softgels** (during the day), and a **Probiotic Defense Formula** capsule (at night, before bed). Drink warm water with 2–4 drops of **lemon** oil and honey to soothe a sore throat and quiet a cough.

DIFFUSE *Protective Blend* or *Cleansing Blend* on-and-off all day in the room where you are resting. A cup of boiling water with a few drops of an essential oil can make a great diffuser in a small space or in your workplace.

> The key to kicking a cold with essential oils is to start using oils when the first symptoms strike and repeating often. Frequent use of oils in rotation will make all the difference; aim for every 30 minutes, if you can.

Your Inner Geek

"Researchers have found that some essential oils--oregano, thyme, and rosewood oils [found in **Grounding Blend**], in particular--create an autolytic (destruction of cells and tissues by enzymes produced by the cells themselves) reaction in organisms, including streptococcus pneumonia." Dr. Diane Horne of Weber State University in Ogden, Utah, to the American Society of Microbiology *Natural News*, 2008.

"The antibacterial activity of essential oils and antibiotics was assessed…[and] the finding highlighted the potential of peppermint, cinnamon bark, and lavender essential oils [to help reduce] usage of antibiotics [and] could be employed as a treatment strategy to decrease the adverse effects and possibly to reverse antibiotic resistance." *Pytomedicine*, 2013.

> A family is a unit composed not only of children but of men, women, an occasional animal, and the common cold. —Ogden Nash

Integrate

Cleaning your home in a "green" way is the best way to avoid colds. Cold germs are adaptogens; so as a synthetic chemical kills them, they regroup and become stronger. Essential oils are also adaptogens; so as the pathogens in nature change, so do the essential oils that kill them. Learn how to keep a clean and green home in the Cleaning section.

Did you know?

This "towel" technique has worked for centuries: add about 2 cups boiling water to a large bowl, and add about 2 to 3 drops each of *eucalyptus* and *Respiratory Blend* to the water. Place a large towel over your head to create a steam tent; close your eyes to avoid eye irritation; and slowly inhale the aroma for 5–10 minutes. Repeat 2–3 times daily until symptoms abate. Adding *lemon*, *thyme*, *rosemary,* or *Protective Blend* can help loosen mucus and heal the throat, nasal passages, and bronchial tubes. Drink plenty of water and unsweetened liquids—tea, broth, kombucha, fresh vegetable juices—when you are sick. Try to avoid simple sugars.

≋ Dive In!

A Sick Day for Amos McGee by Phillip Stead and Erin Stead (Hardcover, 2010).

"Five Surprising Facts About the Common Cold" *Scientific American*, April 15, 2013.

Ah-Choo!: The Uncommon Life of Your Common Cold by Jennifer Ackerman (Hardcover, 2010).

Cheat Sheet

MONTH 1
Protective Softgels
Daily Supplements Pack
Protective Blend
Protective Cleaner
Probiotic Defense Formula
Cleansing Blend
Detoxification Blend

MONTH 2
Respiratory Blend
Invigorating Blend
Daily Supplements Pack
Protective Blend
Probiotic Defense Formula

MONTH 3
Eucalyptus radiata
Daily Supplements Pack
Protective Blend
Protective Hand Wash
Probiotic Defense Formula
Cleansing Blend

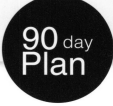

90 day **Plan**

Congestion

Congestion can be caused by a blocking of the nasal passages due to an inflammation of the membranes lining the nose, or it can come from swollen blood vessels in the chest as mucous accumulates.

Our Approach

APPLY warm compresses with *Respiratory Blend*, *frankincense*, *eucalyptus,* or *lavender* over the chest and back. Cover with a warm towel or blanket to keep the body warm. For light nasal congestion, try a *Peppermint Beadlet*.

TRY *Daily Supplements Pack* capsules twice daily with a *GI Cleansing Formula* capsule (during the day) and a *Probiotic Defense Formula* capsule (at night, before bed).

DIFFUSE *Respiratory Blend* or *peppermint* on and off all day in the room where you are resting. A cup of boiling water with a few drops of an essential oil at work can make a great diffuser in a small space.

Your Inner Geek

"*Eucalyptus* oil helps loosen phlegm, so inhaling the vapors may be beneficial for treating bronchitis, coughs, and the flu. Some people apply eucalyptus oil ointments to the nose and chest to relieve sinus and bronchial congestion." University of Maryland Medical Center

"Peppermint's ability to reduce inflammation of nasal passageways has been widely recognized. When menthol vapors are inhaled, nasal passageways are opened to provide temporary relief of nasal and sinus congestion." *AltMD.com*

Apply *Respiratory Blend* to the sinuses on either side of the nose—you get the power of a decongestant and antihistamine without any of the side effects that a drug might cause.

> Both of these botanicals [eucalyptus and sage] act as an excellent remedy for coughs, chest congestion, and sinus infections. I recommend inhaling the steam made from placing eucalyptus and sage [leaves] in boiling water at least 2 times a day. —Dr. Andrew Weil, MD

Integrate

 Congestion relief suggestions in the section on Asthma can help to relieve your symptoms. Drink plenty of water and other fluids, both cold and hot (tea, broth, unsweetened juices), especially if the air in your environment is dry.

Did you know?

There are many ways to clear a stuffy nose naturally. An easy, quick, and inexpensive way to relieve sinus pressure is by alternately thrusting your tongue against the roof of your mouth and then pressing one finger between your eyebrows. This causes the vomer bone, which runs through the nasal passages to the mouth, to rock back and forth, says Lisa DeStefano, DO, an assistant professor at the Michigan State University College of Osteopathic Medicine. The motion loosens the congestion; and after 20 seconds, you'll feel your sinus start to drain.

≋ **Dive In!**

"Gargling with Salt Water Can Ease Cold Symptoms" by Anahad O'Connor, *The New York Times*, September 27, 2010.

"Vital Signs; Nostrums: Seawater Seems to Beat Medicine in Fighting Colds" by Nicholas Bakalar, *The New York Times*, January 22, 2008.

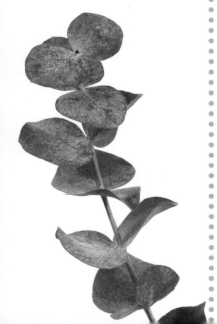

Cheat Sheet

MONTH 1
Respiratory Blend
GI Cleansing Formula
Daily Supplements Pack
Probiotic Defense Formula

MONTH 2
Respiratory Blend
lavender
Daily Supplements Pack
Probiotic Defense Formula
peppermint

MONTH 3
eucalyptus
frankincense
Daily Supplements Pack
Probiotic Defense Formula

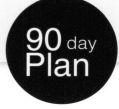

90 day
Plan

Constipation

Constipation refers to bowel movements that are infrequent or hard to pass.

Our Approach

APPLY warm compresses with a drop of *Digestive Blend*, *peppermint*, or *ginger* neat over the abdomen. Use the same oils on the shins, and gently massage up and down for 10 minutes to stimulate digestion. Use a carrier oil like *coconut oil* to make the essential oils easier to massage into the skin.

TRY taking *Daily Supplements Pack* capsules twice daily. You may also want to try 3–4 drops of *Digestive Blend* in a capsule and a *GI Cleansing Formula* capsule (during the day); then take a *Probiotic Defense Formula* capsule (at night, before bed). For persistent constipation, use *Detoxification Complex* for one month. Drink plenty of water, and avoid binding foods like white flour products, sugar, and chocolate. Add *Metabolic Blend* to water, and drink often throughout the day. Eat plenty of fruits and vegetables. Replace one meal each day with a *Trim Shake*.

Your Inner Geek

"Essential fatty acids (such as those found in borage or flax oils)…may also play a role in relieving constipation since the [compounds] they form may help to regulate movement in the bowels." Gene Bruno, Dean of Academics, Huntington College of Health Sciences

Caraway oil found in *Digestive Blend* is warming and stimulating. It is particularly helpful in curing depression and fatigue. It stimulates all the systems and cycles functioning in the body, such as the circulatory system, digestive system, endocrinal secretion system, nervous system, and the excretory system. It can also activate the brain to help keep you awake. *Organic Facts*

Getting into a routine where you drink water regularly throughout the day may help alleviate constipation. This is especially true of the elderly, who tend to lose their ability to feel thirsty as they age.

An elderly lady went to her doctor to see what could be done about her constipation. "It's terrible," she said, "I haven't moved my bowels in a week." "I see. Have you done anything about it?" asked the doctor. "Naturally," she replied, "I sit in the bathroom for a half-hour in the morning and again at night." "No," the doctor said, "I mean do you take anything?" "Naturally," she answered, "I take a book."

Integrate

The "clean eating" program found in the 90-Day Plan Cheat Sheet in the Weight Management section can help you maintain a healthy weight and help you to release toxins from your body (which may not be occurring properly if you are suffering from constipation).

Did you know?

Constipation is caused by many factors and can lead to other more serious ailments, even in children. Do not be afraid to talk to your doctor about irregularity. Bowel movements should occur at least once a day and should be passed without strain.

If you find you develop hemorrhoids, take a few drops of **cypress** diluted with **coconut oil,** and gently apply it to the affected area to reduce pain and swelling.

≋ Dive In!

The Ins and Outs of Poop, A Guide to Treating Childhood Constipation by Thomas R. Duhamel (Paperback, 2012).

Everyone Poops by Taro Gomi (Hardcover, 2004).

"Natural Constipation Relief Strategies You Should Know About" by Dr. Joseph Mercola, *mercola.com* April 11, 2009.

"Elevate your feet for better elimination" *SquattyPotty.com.*

Cheat Sheet

MONTH 1
cypress
Digestive Blend
coconut oil
ginger
Daily Supplements Pack
peppermint

MONTH 2
GI Cleansing Formula
Daily Supplements Pack
Probiotic Defense Formula
Metabolic Blend

MONTH 3
Digestive Blend
Daily Supplements Pack
Probiotic Defense Formula
Trim Shake
Detoxification Blend

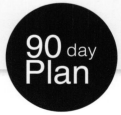

90 day
Plan

Cough

We all know how painful and disruptive a cough can be. Some are dry, others wet; some can be productive; others will cause a spasm that seems never to end. You may need to try 2 or 3 oils to find the right combination for relief.

Our Approach

APPLY warm compresses with *eucalyptus*, *frankincense*, or *lavender* neat over the chest and back. For a severe cough, also apply to the soles of the feet. Follow this with *Respiratory Blend* neat. Apply 1 drop *peppermint* (dilute for sensitive skin) on top to drive in the other oils. Cover with a warm towel or blanket to keep the body warm. See the Congestion section for another "towel method."

TRY *Daily Supplements Pack* and *GI Cleansing Formula* capsules (during the day) and a *Probiotic Defense Formula* capsule (at night before bed). One drop of *peppermint* or *lemon* oil on a spoon with honey or raw agave syrup can make a quick throat soother and tastes like a lemon drop candy. Take *Protective Throat Drops* with you to help quiet your cough during the day.

DIFFUSE *Respiratory Blend* or *peppermint* on-and-off during the day in the room where you are resting. A cup of boiling water with a few drops of an essential oil at work can make a great diffuser in a small space.

Comparing and reviewing 25 studies on over-the-counter cough medicine, a recent research review published in The Cochrane Library, an online collection of healthcare databases, determined that there is no good evidence for or against the effectiveness of formulas such as Robitussin® and Mucinex®.

Your Inner Geek

"Essential oils are used in aromatherapy to treat a cough in two general ways: by rubbing the oil on your chest or by inhaling the fumes of the oil. In the first approach, a few drops of the essential oil are mixed with a small amount of a carrier oil. The mixture is then rubbed on the chest to relieve a cough." *AltMD.com*

"*Eucalyptus* is a standard ingredient in cough drops and cough syrups, as well as in oils added to humidifiers. A standardized combination of eucalyptus oil plus two other essential oils has been studied for effectiveness in a variety of respiratory conditions. [With the most effective] combination therapy containing cineole from eucalyptus, d- limonene from citrus fruit, and alpha-pinene from pine."
NYU Langone Medical Center.

> **Doctor: Your cough sounds much better today.**
> **Patient: It should. I've been practicing all night.**

Integrate

The 90-Day Plan Cheat Sheet for Colds is your complete guide to dealing with all your cold symptoms, including the worst coughs. If you can stop the early symptoms like a runny nose or post nasal drip, you may be able to avoid a cough from developing. If your cold tends to start with a cough, learn how to keep your lungs strong all year long.

Did you know?

We think most will agree, nighttime can be the worst enemy of a person with a cough. Getting to sleep and staying asleep can be the difference between getting better and staying sick. Be sure to diffuse **Respiratory Blend** in the bedroom at least 1 hour before sleep to set up an environment of relaxed respiration in addition to using your oils for cough and sleep. We like *lavender* on the soles of the feet and *eucalyptus* on the chest and back. Need something stronger? Apply **Respiratory Blend** and **Soothing Blend** to the chest, back, and spine. Sucking on an **Protective Throat Drop** can also help.

≋ Dive In!

Aromatherapy for the Healthy Child: More Than 300 Natural, Nontoxic and Fragrant Essential Oil Blends by Valerie Ann Worwood (Paperback 2000).

"Is Honey More Effective Than Cough Medicine?" by Dr. Joseph Mercola, mercola.com December 22, 2007.

Cheat Sheet

MONTH 1
Respiratory Blend
GI Cleansing Formula
Probiotic Defense Formula
lavender
Daily Supplements Pack
Protective Throat Drops

MONTH 2
Respiratory Blend
lemon
Daily Supplements Pack
peppermint
Probiotic Defense Formula

MONTH 3
Soothing Blend
eucalyptus
frankincense
Daily Supplements Pack
Probiotic Defense Formula

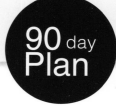

90 day **Plan**

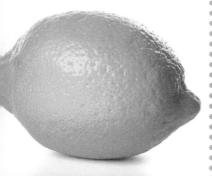

Cuts, Scrapes & Bruises

Whether dealing with a cut, scrape, or bruise, the first line of attack must be to prevent infection and the second to heal the skin quickly without scarring.

Our Approach

APPLY *Grounding Blend* around the area to help with pain, bruising, and swelling, after using a clean, warm cloth to remove any debris. Spritz with **lavender** mixed with water and organic aloe, and apply **frankincense** topically, covering if necessary. Once the wound is closed, apply **lavender**, **frankincense,** and **helichrysum** to prevent scarring. Apply **cypress** to the bottoms of the feet to help speed healing.

TRY *Essential Oil Cellular Complex* capsules or liquid complex (internally) to promote healing of the skin.

DIFFUSE *Calming Blend* if you have trouble sleeping or if you are shaken from the trauma.

Using a "triple antibiotic" cream for minor cuts is like using a sledgehammer to crack a walnut. A simpler alternative, **melaleuca**, can be applied straight to the skin and is a natural antiseptic, antibacterial and germicide, fungicide. *Journal of Hospital Infection*

Your Inner Geek

For wound treatment, "You can dilute your essential oil in a carrier oil, which can be almost any type of vegetable oil. The rule of thumb for dilution is to every 2 tablespoons of carrier oil add 15 drops of essential oil from a dropper. This will give you a 2.5 percent dilution. You can use slightly more concentrated oil if you are applying it to a small, localized area of the body. Once you make this healing mixture, you should use it on the injured area several times a day.

"There is much scientific literature that documents the antiseptic activity of essential oils but limited studies examining the use of essential oils on the skin to prevent infection and heal wounds. Several small studies have found benefits to lavender, tea tree and chamomile essential oils."
AltMD.com

> **Failures are like skinned knees; painful but superficial.**
> **—Carl Sandburg**

Integrate

Kids get into a lot of "scrapes." Getting oils on the body as soon as possible is key. Be sure to carry your first aid oils with you so that you always have what you need. Adhesive strips will not stick to the skin once essential oils are applied. Apply a gauze pad, or allow the skin to dry before covering with a small bandage.

Did you know?

The injury required to produce a bruise varies with age. While it may take quite a bit of force to cause a bruise in a young child, even minor bumps and scrapes may cause extensive bruising or ecchymosis in an elderly person. Blood vessels become more fragile as we age, and bruising may even occur without prior injury in the elderly. The amount of bruising may also be affected by medications. Do your homework and be sure to understand how your medications may affect you.

Dive In!

Cuts, Scrapes, Scabs and Scars by Alvin Silverstein, Virginia Silverstein, and Laura Silverstein Nunn (Paperback, 2000).

Everything First Aid Book: How to Handle Falls and Breaks, Choking, Cuts and Scrapes, Insect Bites and Rashes, Burns, Poisoning, and When to Call 911 (Everything Series) by Nadine Saubers, RN (Paperback, 2008).

Cheat Sheet

MONTH 1
Grounding Blend
Essential Oil Cellular
Complex
frankincense
lavender
melaleuca

MONTH 2
cypress
Essential Oil Cellular
Complex
helichrysum

MONTH 3
Grounding Blend
Essential Oil Cellular
Complex
Calming Blend

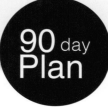

90 day
Plan

Dental Health

Dental health reaches beyond just your teeth and gums. Maintain the health of your mouth, teeth, gums, tongue, and throat, to insure good dental and overall health.

Our Approach

APPLY *Protective Blend* and *frankincense* to gums 1–4 times a month. *Protective Blend* is also great for mild toothaches and infections. Brush daily with *Protective Toothpaste*. If you are experiencing dental pain, apply *Soothing Blend* along the jawline when needed. Place a *Peppermint Beadlet* between the gums and an aching tooth to temporarily relieve minor tooth discomfort.

TRY *Daily Supplements Pack* capsules to support dental health. Before every meal, take *Digestive Enzyme Complex* capsules for better digestion.

DIFFUSE *Calming Blend* before your visit to the dentist to calm any nervous tension you may be feeling.

Experiencing tooth pain? Try a drop of *clove* or *Protective Blend* on a cotton swab, and apply it around the affected tooth. Placing the oil on dental floss and gently (we know it hurts!) flossing will get the oil down into the crevasses. For pain, try a mouth rinse with one or 2 drops of *clove* or *Protective Blend* in 4–6 ounces of water.

Your Inner Geek

"In 1923, Dr. Weston Price, the chairman of the research section of the ADA, recommended thymol (in clove oil) for sterilization in root canal therapy. In 1938, the 'Accepted Dental Remedies' of the ADA stated that the antiseptic efficiency of thymol was higher than that of phenol as a canal filling material and for direct pulp capping."
Dentistry Today, 2003.

"Studies have confirmed that for patients with gingivitis, who brush and floss routinely, the adjunctive use of an essential oil containing an essential oil mouth rinse provides a clinically significant and meaningful additional benefit in reducing plaque and gingivitis."
American Dental Association, 2004.

Integrate

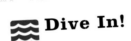 Clean eating is one way to improve your dental health. Avoiding sticky and processed foods will lower the acidity in your body and keep teeth strong. Replace these foods with fat burning foods that also protect your teeth, and you will get a double bonus! Try our easy program in the 90-Day Plan Cheat Sheet in the Weight Management section. Our social media sites provide you with great meal suggestions and other clean eating resources.

Did you know?

Dating back as far as 220 B.C., *clove* oil was commonly used to freshen breath. During the time of the Renaissance, cloves were part of a more hands-on approach to oral care. Cloves were used for their antiseptic qualities and in the treatment and prevention of plaque. Avicenna, who was the teacher of Hippocrates, also made use of *clove* oil in pill form to treat rotting teeth and gums.

≋ Dive In!

"Reversing Gum Disease Naturally" by Sandra Senzon, *New York Times*, April 25 2003

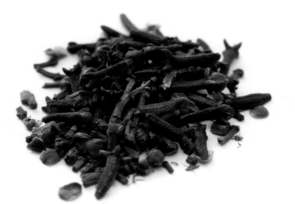

Cheat Sheet

MONTH 1
clove
Protective Toothpaste
Daily Supplements Pack
Calming Blend
Digestive Enzyme
Complex

MONTH 2
Soothing Blend
Daily Supplements Pack
Protective Blend
Digestive Enzyme
Complex

MONTH 3
frankincense
Daily Supplements Pack
Digestive Enzyme
Complex

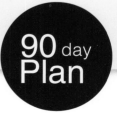

90 day
Plan

Depression

Depression affects one out of every three Americans and, unfortunately, is rising every year. Medications may have a temporary effect, but they are also associated with many unpleasant side effects.

 ## Our Approach

APPLY *Joyful Blend* and *Grounding Blend* 2–3 times a day over the heart, on the wrists, and on the feet.

TRY *Daily Supplements Pack* capsules 2 times a day. Take *Digestive Enzyme Complex* and *Probiotic Defense Formula* capsules with every meal.

DIFFUSE *Invigorating Blend* to uplift or *Calming Blend* to relax.

Eliminating sugars and processed food from your diet can help end feelings of lethargy and despair. Although high carbohydrate foods like muffins, crackers, and cakes can be comforting initially, they play havoc with your blood sugar levels and can leave you feeling tired and sad soon after eating them.

Your Inner Geek

Massage therapy with essential oils may benefit people with depression. The scents are thought by some to stimulate positive emotions in the area of the brain responsible for memories and emotions, but the benefits seem to be related to relaxation caused by the scents and the massage. A person's belief that the treatment will help also influences whether it works. University of Maryland Medical Center

A 2005 article by Stephen Warrenburg in *Chemical Senses* studied the effect of essential oils on mood: 44.6% of study participants found vanilla relaxing while 27.2% reported feelings of happiness.

> ## Sadness is but a wall between two gardens.
> ### —Kahlil Gibran

Integrate

 The 90-Day Plan Cheat Sheet is written for those with any degree of anxiety or depression. Although this is a 90-day plan, it can be used on an ongoing basis until you feel like your emotions have leveled. Each person's chemistry is different. The amount of time you will need to get your body balanced can vary. Use the products for at least 90 days, and then slowly decrease the amount of product you are using to find the level that you need to keep your body balanced.

Did you know?

Taking two **Food Nutrient Complex** capsules twice a day (part of the **Daily Supplements Pack**) is a great way to get the B vitamins you need, and almost all of the vitamins in the B group play an active role in tackling depression. According to a study done in 1986, "Vitamin B1 (thiamin) and B2 (riboflavin) deficiencies have been linked to depression; while vitamin B3 (niacin) has been used to treat depression because it can increase serotonin levels. Serotonin is a neurotransmitter that helps relay messages from one side of the brain to the other. Without it, it can be hard to balance our mood."
A Biochemical and Neuroendocrine Study of the Serotonergic System in Depression

We've all heard about the benefits of taking an omega-3 supplement if fighting depression. In 2009, the American College of Nutrition found that there may be important differences depending on the type of omega-3 supplement. Fish oil contains two types: DHA (docosahexaenoic acid) and EPA (eicosapentaenoic acid).

Studies that used pure DHA or more than 50% DHA reported no effect on depression. Studies that used pure EPA or more than 50% EPA found that symptoms improved—which is exactly what's in **Essential Oil Omega Complex**—our personal favorite.

Cheat Sheet

MONTH 1
Grounding Blend
Joyful Blend
Daily Supplements Pack
Digestive Enzyme
Complex

MONTH 2
Daily Supplements Pack
Calming Blend
Digestive Enzyme
Complex

MONTH 3
Invigorating Blend
Daily Supplements Pack
Digestive Enzyme
Complex

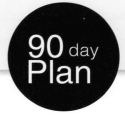

≋ Dive In!

Happiness by Joan Chittister (Paperback, 2011).

Sustainable Wellness: An Integrative Approach to Transform Your Mind, Body, and Spirit Matt Mumber by Heather Reed and Andrew Weil (Paperback, 2012).

"Are Probiotics the New Prozac?" by Dr. Joseph Mercola, *mercola.com*, July 25, 2013.

Diabetes

Diabetes is a disease in which your blood glucose (also called blood sugar) levels are too high. Glucose comes from the foods we eat. Insulin is a hormone that helps the glucose get into your cells to give them energy. With Type 1 diabetes, your body does not make insulin. With Type 2 diabetes, the more common type, the body does not use insulin well, causing the glucose to stay in the blood instead of going into cells where it is needed.

Our Approach

APPLY *Digestive Blend* and *fennel* neat to the soles of the feet, 2 times daily.

TRY 1–2 drops of *cassia* under the tongue before meals. For sugar cravings, try 1 drop of *clove* on the tip of the tongue. To promote healthy eating, try *Daily Supplements Pack* capsules, and substitute one meal a day with a *Trim Shake*. Take *Digestive Enzyme Complex* capsules before each meal to help improve digestion, blood sugar balance, and nutrient absorption.

DIFFUSE *peppermint* to clear the mind and reduce cravings.

Carry *cassia* or *cinnamon* (both in the cinnamon family) with you. *Cinnamon* has been shown to help regulate blood sugar levels. Take 1–2 drops of either of these oils under the tongue before eating to help regulate blood sugar.

Your Inner Geek

In a study featured in the 2008 issue of *Asia Pacific Journal of Clinical Nutrition*, "Fennel and a few other herbs and vegetables commonly used in Indian cuisine showed significant inhibitory effects on the negative activity of (aldose reductase) an enzyme involved in the conversion of glucose. The authors believe that including fennel, as well as spinach, cumin, lemon, basil and black pepper in a diet, may help manage diabetic complications."

According to the World Health Organization (WHO) in 2013, approximately 150 million people worldwide have type 2 diabetes, and it is a growing health concern.

> ## I know of no other disease that's increasing at [about] 8% per year.
> ### —Dr. John Anderson, MD, American Diabetes Association

Integrate

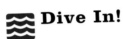 Clinical trials have shown that losing just 5 to 7 percent of body weight—that's 10 to 14 pounds for a 200-pound person—and getting at least 150 minutes of moderate physical activity each week (about 20 minutes a day) reduces the risk of type 2 diabetes by nearly 60 percent in those at high risk for developing the disease! *Centers for Disease Control (CDC)*. Try our easy program in the 90-Day Plan Cheat Sheet in the Weight Management section, and visit our social media sites for fat-burning information on foods, oils, and supplements.

Did you know?

The CDC estimates that as many as 1 in 3 U.S. adults could have diabetes by 2050 if current trends continue. Type 2 diabetes, in which the body gradually loses its ability to use insulin properly, accounts for 90% to 95% of cases.

≋ Dive In!

"Are Contaminants Silencing Our Genes?" by Bette Hileman and Environmental Health News, *Scientific American*. August 3, 2009. Some chemicals may leave people vulnerable to diseases like cancer and diabetes, not by mutating genes but by turning them off or on at the wrong time.

The End of Diabetes: The Eat to Live Plan to Prevent and Reverse Diabetes by Joel Fuhrman (Paperback, 2012).

Fast Food Nation: The Dark Side of the All-American Meal by Eric Schlosser (Paperback, 2012).

Forks Over Knives by T. Colin Campbell and Caldwell B. Esselstyn Jr. (Movie, 2011).

Cheat Sheet

MONTH 1
cinnamon
Digestive Blend
fennel
Daily Supplements Pack
Digestive Enzyme Complex

MONTH 2
cassia
Digestive Blend
Daily Supplements Pack
Digestive Enzyme Complex
Trim Shake

MONTH 3
clove
Digestive Blend
Daily Supplements Pack
peppermint
Digestive Enzyme Complex

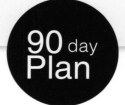

90 day **Plan**

Diarrhea

No matter the cause, the biggest threat to the body from diarrhea is dehydration. Keeping liquids in the body is key to the healing process. Oils and supplements can help play an important role in keeping the body from dehydrating.

Our Approach

APPLY 2 drops of *Digestive Blend* neat to the abdomen, and massage it in a gentle circular motion. Apply often at first and then consistently every 2–4 hours for at least 24 hours after the diarrhea has subsided.

TRY 1 drop of *peppermint* or *ginger* in water or *Digestive Softgels* until diarrhea has subsided. To improve immunity against pathogens that lead to diarrhea, take 1 drop of *oregano* in a capsule daily, and continue for a week after the diarrhea has subsided. Then, take *Daily Supplements Pack* capsules to help restore nutrition and *Probiotic Defense Formula* to help restore proper intestinal flora. Drink water with *lemon* in small doses to help replace what has been lost.

DIFFUSE *peppermint* to settle the stomach.

"Your digestive tract is a delicate ecosystem of both good and bad bacteria," says David Rakel, MD. "When you eat a lot of processed food or take antibiotics, you can wipe out these 'friendly' bacteria. This allows the bad guys to take over, leading to IBS, diarrhea, and other problems." Maintaining a healthy balance of bacteria is easier when you take a probiotic supplement that includes a lot of good bacteria like *Probiotic Defense Formula* capsules.

Your Inner Geek

Diarrhea caused by contaminated food or water is a frequent problem for travelers. Up to 10% of people who get diarrhea while traveling end up developing persistent diarrhea—but probiotics may help. A 2007 report concluded that probiotics lowered the risk of getting travelers' diarrhea and that the strongest evidence pointed to benefits from L. acidophilus and B. bifidum" [both found in *Probiotic Defense Formula*]. WebMD

Taking caraway oil [found in *Digestive Blend*] as part of a specific combination with *peppermint* oil seems to relieve heartburn, including symptoms of fullness and mild gastrointestinal spasms, like those associated with diarrhea.
WebMD

> **It is still just unbelievable to us that diarrhea is one of the leading causes of child deaths in the world.—Melinda Gates**

Integrate

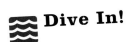 The 90-Day Plan Cheat Sheet for Colds has a complete guide to symptom relief for all your needs. This easy-to-follow symptom relief guide will provide all the direction you need to use your products effectively. Remember to keep these commonly needed products on hand so that you have them when a diarrhea strikes!

Did you know?

Manage stress—that feeling of butterflies in your stomach has a physiological basis. "There's a lot of cross talk between the brain and the gut," explains James Mullin, PhD, a clinical neuropsychologist. Your GI tract has its own nervous system, which is why stress can cause digestive problems such as diarrhea, heartburn, and irritable bowel syndrome (IBS). Learn to manage stress—and reduce GI problems—by exploring massage, art therapy, breathing exercises, and other relaxation techniques.

Dive In!

"Drier Climate May Spread Diarrhea" by Alex Kirby and The Daily Climate, *Scientific American*, March 28, 2013. Researchers say they have found a clear link between climate change and the spread of diarrhea and similar diseases in one African country. But the nature of the link may be unexpected.

Healthy Digestion the Natural Way: Preventing and Healing Heartburn, Constipation, Gas, Diarrhea, Inflammatory Bowel and Gallbladder Diseases, Ulcers, Irritable Bowel Syndrome and More by D. Lindsey Berkson (Paperback, 2000).

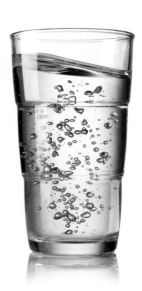

Cheat Sheet

MONTH 1
Digestive Blend
Digestive Softgels
Daily Supplements Pack
oregano
Probiotic Defense Formula
Digestive Enzyme
Complex

MONTH 2
Daily Supplements Pack
peppermint
Probiotic Defense Formula
Digestive Enzyme
Complex

MONTH 3
ginger
Probiotic Defense Formula
Daily Supplements Pack
Digestive Enzyme
Complex

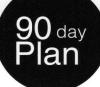

90 day **Plan**

Digestion

Digestive issues run the gamut from an upset stomach after overeating or eating the wrong foods to a serious chronic disorder such as Crohn's Disease or Irritable Bowel Syndrome and chronic constipation.

Our Approach

APPLY 2 drops of *Digestive Blend*, *ginger,* or *peppermint* (dilute for sensitive skin) on the abdomen on a daily basis (more often if problems are severe). Use *Calming Blend* to reduce the stress of a chronic disorder.

TRY *Digestive Enzyme Complex* capsules with meals to help promote proper digestion and increase nutritional absorption. Try *Probiotic Defense Formula* capsules at night to promote good digestion and healthy bowel movements. Take *Digestive Enzyme Complex* capsules between meals to break down toxins in the digestive tract. Take *Daily Supplements Pack* capsules twice daily to help support proper nutrition.

DIFFUSE *Calming Blend* day and night to help reduce overall stress and lessen the stress on the digestive tract.

Dr. Andrew Weil says, "Try plant-derived digestive enzymes that can help digest specific nutrients. Those containing amylase can help with carbohydrate digestion, those with lipase are for fats, protease for protein, lactase for dairy products, and cellulose for fiber." [Our new favorite enzyme complex (which contains all four) is *Digestive Enzyme Complex*.]

Your Inner Geek

"Any of us who've had a meal and felt bloated and full afterwards knows what it's like to suffer from poor digestion. Sadly, so much of what's in today's complex food is nearly indigestible or outright bad for you. In fact, even when your digestive enzymes are flowing freely and in the right amounts, they may only be able to break down and extract about 40 to 50 percent of your food's true nutrient value. And the more refined and processed a food is, the lower your gut's capacity to retrieve what's there and distribute it to your body. Your digestive organs and enzymes end up working overtime, especially if you regularly eat more than you should. This not only takes a toll on our digestive system, but it also short changes your immune system.

"As a result of understanding the critical connection between the gut and immunity, I'm fully convinced

Cheat Sheet

that nobody can achieve optimum health without focusing on the health of their gut. A simple approach to maintaining a healthy gut is the use of supplemental enzymes."
Dr. Mehmet Oz

Integrate

Regularly applying, ingesting, and diffusing essential oils can help with good digestion. The slow and steady use of oils, supplements, and probiotics will help to rebuild a strong and healthy digestive system.

Did you know?

Ulcers can be caused by diet, stress, or pathogens. No matter what the cause, bringing the digestive system into proper balance should help symptoms caused by ulcers and other stomach ailments such as reflux and flatulence. Eating a diet full of vegetables, fruits, and other enzyme-rich foods helps to promote proper digestion. Try blending or juicing fresh foods into smoothies and soups if you find them hard to digest. **Probiotic Defense Formula** capsules at night will help replenish good bacteria in the gut. **Digestive Enzyme Complex** will help digest foods more completely. **Calming Blend** used daily will help to keep stress from attacking the digestive system.

Fermented foods (like pickles, kimchi, sauerkraut, kvass, or miso) have been shown to be beneficial for a number of health conditions including candida overgrowth, IBS and digestive difficulties, sugar/carb cravings, and other inflammatory disorders. What's more, science is starting to show that our modern lifestyle of completely eschewing bacteria with pasteurized foods, hand sanitizers, disinfectants, and antibiotics is actually making us more, not less, susceptible to illness and allergies. Regular inclusion of fermented foods in the diet naturally combats bad bacteria and strengthens the immune system.

Dive In!

Fermented Foods for Health: Use the Power of Probiotic Foods to Improve Your Digestion, Strengthen Your Immunity, and Prevent Illness by Deirdre Rawlings (Paperback, 2013).

Digestive Wellness: Strengthen the Immune System and Prevent Disease Through Healthy Digestion, Fourth Edition by Elizabeth Lipski (Paperback, 2011).

"Preserving Plenty: The Beauty of Fermented Foods" by Sarah Dickerman, *Saveur Magazine*, May 16, 2013. The process of fermentation is the secret behind some of the world's most delicious foods.

MONTH 1
Digestive Blend
Probiotic Defense Formula
Daily Supplements Pack
Digestive Enzyme Complex

MONTH 2
peppermint
Probiotic Defense Formula
Daily Supplements Pack
Calming Blend
Digestive Enzyme Complex

MONTH 3
ginger
Probiotic Defense Formula
Daily Supplements Pack
Digestive Enzyme Complex

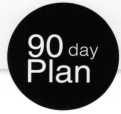

90 day Plan

Earaches

Although most common in children, earaches can occur at any age. Earaches are often caused by inflammation, dehydration, or an over proliferation of pathogens, and pain can range from minor to debilitating. "People think earwax is dirt. It's not dirt. It's a protective coating for our ear canal."
Dr. Rick Friedman, Neurologist, House Clinic, Los Angeles.

Our Approach

APPLY *Tension Blend* roll-on and *Grounding Blend* around the ear (never in). Dilute these with *coconut oil* if the skin around the ear becomes red or irritated.

TRY *Daily Supplements Pack* capsules, and take a *Protective Softgel* during the day and a *Probiotic Defense Formula* capsule at night. Drinking water with *lemon* or *Invigorating Blend* will help to flush out toxins.

DIFFUSE *lavender* for its germ fighting and relaxing qualities and to settle the stomach.

Your Inner Geek

 Applying certain essential oils to the (outer) ear canal appears to be an effective treatment for acute otitis media (middle ear infection), according to a recent animal study at Landspitali University Hospital in Reykjavik, Iceland. Vapors released by essential oils, such as basil, have produced rapid bactericidal (antibacterial) effects as they diffuse into the middle ear. Treatment with basil oil "cured or healed 56% to 81% of rats… [and] placebo cure rates did not exceed 6%."
American Speech-Language-Hearing Association

Apply
Soothing Blend roll-on around the ear to lessen the pain and reduce swelling. Essential oils can help diminish pain safely. Never pour essential oils into the ear!

> **Praise does wonders for our sense of hearing**
> **—Arnold Glasgow**

Integrate

Whether focusing on symptom relief or working on the root cause, an easy application of oils can do wonders to relieve an earache. Be sure to apply often. Many times people do not get the results they desire because they are not using their oils often enough. Don't be afraid to use your oils every 20 minutes the first day.

Did you know?

The ears are fragile instruments. Damage to this delicate apparatus results from both volume and length of exposure to sound. Very loud noises, or chronic exposure to sound even when it is not particularly loud, can wreak havoc on our present and future ability to hear.

Even toys meant for young children can generate ear-damaging levels of noise. The American Speech-Language-Hearing Association lists as potential hazards cap guns, talking dolls, vehicles with horns and sirens, walkie-talkies, rubber squeaky toys, musical instruments and toys with cranks, earbuds, and headsets. According to the association, some toy sirens and squeaky rubber toys can emit sounds of 90 dB, as loud as a lawn mower.

The Association suggests that parents with normal hearing test new toys before giving them to a child. "If the toy sounds loud, don't buy it." For noisy toys already bought, consider removing the batteries or taping over the speaker.

As for headphones, A good plan is to set a maximum volume while in a quiet environment and never go above that.

 ## Dive In!

"Ear Infections Too Often Misdiagnosed, Then Overtreated" by Laurie Tarkan, *New York Times*, February 12, 2008.

"Obesity's Tie to Childhood Earaches" by Melinda Wenner, *Scientific American*, December 9, 2008.

"Shouting Won't Help: Why I - and 50 million Other Americans - Can't Hear You" by Katherine Bouton (Paperback 2013).

Cheat Sheet

MONTH 1
GI Cleansing Formula
Daily Supplements Pack
Protective Softgel
Tension Blend
Probiotic Defense Formula

MONTH 2
Grounding Blend
lemon
Daily Supplements Pack
Probiotic Defense Formula

MONTH 3
Invigorating Blend
coconut oil
Daily Supplements Pack
Probiotic Defense Formula

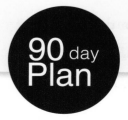

90 day **Plan**

Energy

Energy comes from the body's ability to process what we eat and turn it into energy we can use. When we eat foods our body cannot process, we can end up being tired and sluggish. This can lead to sleepless nights, which compound exhaustion. Once run down, we are vulnerable to illness, which can weaken us further.

Our Approach

APPLY a few drops of *peppermint*, *black pepper*, and/or *basil* to the back of the neck for a great pick-me-up.

TRY a *Daily Supplements Pack* twice daily to promote good nutrition and a healthy metabolism, and try a *Digestive Enzyme Complex* with meals. For lasting energy, try a drop each of *grapefruit*, *fennel*, and *black pepper* in a capsule for an energy boost. For an extra boost, try an *Energy & Stamina Complex* with your biggest meals for sustained energy, stamina, and endurance. (This is great for athletes, workaholics, and busy moms!)

DIFFUSE *peppermint* or *lemon* in a room where you are working. This can help keep your energy high and your mind alert.

Your Inner Geek

A team of researchers led by Bruce N. Ames, professor of molecular and cell biology at UC Berkeley, fed older rats two chemicals normally found in the body's cells and available as dietary supplements: acetyl-L-carnitine and an antioxidant, alpha-lipoic acid [found in *Energy & Stamina Complex*]. In 3 articles published in 2002 in Proceedings of the National Academy of Sciences, Ames and his colleagues report the surprising results: Not only did the older rats do better on memory tests, but they also had more pep, and the energy-producing organelles

For an instant energy boost, drop out of your busy life for 10 minutes and hit the road, or the hallways of your office. Walking is an energizer. Even a 10-minute walk can help you overcome feelings of fatigue. And yes, it works better than a sugar infusion. In a study published two decades ago but still often-quoted, Robert Thayer, PhD, professor at California State University, Long Beach, compared the energizing effects on 12 different days when 18 people either ate a candy bar or walked briskly for 10 minutes. Walking was the better bet. Walking increased energy for two hours. The sugar snack initially boosted energy, but after an hour, participants were more tired and had less energy.

in their cells worked better.

"With the two supplements together, these old rats got up and did the Macarena," said Ames, also a researcher at Children's Hospital Oakland Research Institute. "The brain looks better, they are full of energy—everything we looked at looks more like a young animal." University of California, Berkeley

Integrate

Treat yourself to a massage to help detoxification. No matter what may be off balance in your body, an **Aroma Massage** treatment can jump-start your system and give your body a boost of energy. Following the 90-Day Plan Cheat Sheet in the Nutrition section can give you the support you need to continue your detox and reach the energy level you desire.

Did you know?

High-intensity interval training has also been shown to produce greater health benefits overall than conventional aerobic training. A recent study found doing just three minutes of high intensity training per week for four weeks could lead to significant changes in important health indices, including a 24 percent improvement in insulin sensitivity.

Another important benefit of high-intensity interval training is its ability to naturally increase your body's production of human growth hormone (HGH), also known as "the fitness hormone." HGH is a synergistic, foundational biochemical underpinning that promotes muscle and effectively burns excessive fat. It also plays an important part in promoting overall health and longevity. This is something you cannot easily get from conventional aerobic endurance training (Dr. Joseph Mercola).

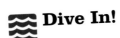 **Dive In!**

"Energy Shot's 'No Crash' Claim Is Disputed by Watchdog" by Barry Meier, *The New York Times*, January 2, 2013.

How to Boost Your Energy: 55 Amazing Truths about Nutrition, Exercise, Sleep, Life Organization and Stress Relief That Will Keep You Energized All Day by Paul Clements (E-book, 2012).

Cheat Sheet

MONTH 1
black pepper
Daily Supplements Pack
Energy & Stamina Complex
Digestive Enzyme Complex

MONTH 2
fennel
grapefruit
Daily Supplements Pack
Energy & Stamina Complex

MONTH 3
basil
Daily Supplements Pack
Energy & Stamina Complex
peppermint

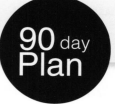

90 day **Plan**

Feet, Hands, & Nails

The eyes are the windows to the soul, but the hands, nails, and feet are the measure of age. You can hide your age almost everywhere else, but your hands, nails, and feet will usually give you away. A true indicator of improving health is the appearance of your feet, hands, and nails.

Our Approach

APPLY *Invigorating Scrub* once a week to wash hands and feet. Moisturize cuticles and nails with **Rose Oil Hand Lotion** and **myrrh**. Mix **cypress** in **Hand & Body Lotion,** and apply the mixture to the feet to improve circulation. Mix **Grounding Blend** into an organic ointment to soften and heal callouses.

TRY *Daily Supplements Pack* capsules daily. Fish oils have long been touted as a beauty secret for great hands and nails.

DIFFUSE *lavender* or *frankincense* at night. The calming effects of these oils are very supportive of hand and feet health.

For warts and fungal issues, apply *oregano*, *melaleuca*, *lemongrass*, and/or *Protective Blend* to the area, cover with cotton, and wrap with plastic wrap to create an airtight seal. Repeat twice a day for up to 6 weeks.

Your Inner Geek

According to Valerie Ann Worwood, author of *The Complete Book of Essential Oils & Aromatherapy*, several essential oils prevent over-drying of the nails and cuticles and protect them from environmental damage. Always mix essential oils into a base oil such as fractionated coconut oil to add extra emollients. Worwood says essential oils such as **cypress** and **eucalyptus** help maintain the moisture balance in the nail. *Grapefruit*, *lavender*, and **lemon** provide healing from environmental irritants. *Peppermint* and *rosemary* act as stimulants and promote blood flow to the nail bed. You can use these oils individually or blend several drops of each into a base oil.

Integrate

Summer is a great time to start taking care of your hands and feet. Everyone wants to put their best foot forward, especially in sandals. Follow us on social media for tips on how to care for your hands, nails, and feet in the summer and all year long!

Did you know?

Americans spent a whopping $33.3 billion on cosmetics and other beauty products in 2010, according to the Commerce Department. That's more than consumers shelled out to buy new foreign cars ($27 billion) or TVs ($25 billion).

〰 Dive In!

A Consumer's Dictionary of Cosmetic Ingredients 7th Edition: Complete Information About the Harmful and Desirable Ingredients Found in Cosmetics and Cosmeceuticals by Ruth Winter (Paperback, 2009).

No More Dirty Looks: The Truth about Your Beauty Products—and the Ultimate Guide to Safe and Clean Cosmetics by Siobhan O'Connor and Alexandra Spunt (Paperback, 2010).

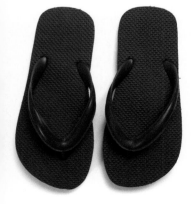

Cheat Sheet

MONTH 1
myrrh
Invigorating Scrub
Rose Oil Hand Lotion
Daily Supplements Pack

MONTH 2
Grounding Blend
peppermint
Hand & Body Lotion
Daily Supplements Pack

MONTH 3
Protective Blend
cypress
frankincense
Daily Supplements Pack

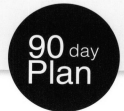

90 day Plan

Fever

A fever is an elevation of body temperature. This happens when the body is trying to kill off a pathogen. If a fever increases or is sustained for a prolonged period of time, it is important to seek medical attention right away.

Our Approach

APPLY A few drops of *lavender*, *peppermint*, and *lemon*, to the back of the neck and on the bottoms of the feet every 10–20 minutes until the fever subsides.

TRY *GI Cleansing Formula* and a *Probiotic Defense Formula* capsules during and at least 2 weeks after a fever has subsided. Rebuild your strength by taking *Daily Supplements Pack* capsules twice daily.

DIFFUSE *Calming Blend* or *lavender* to help you sleep and recover.

Remember to drink plenty of water and eat lightly when feeling feverish. This gives the body extra support to fight illness and recover quickly.

Your Inner Geek

 "Medicinal plants have been used widely to treat a variety of vector ailments [associated with high fevers] such as malaria. The demand for plant-based medicines is growing, as they are generally considered to be safer, non-toxic, and less harmful than synthetic drugs. This article reviews potential anti-dengue activities from plants distributed around the world…Crude extracts and essential oils obtained from 31 species showed a broad activity against Flavivirus. Current studies show that natural products represent a rich potential source of new anti-dengue compounds." Universiti Teknologi Malaysia, 2013

The result obtained in this study goes a long way in validating the ethnobotanical usage of these medicinal plants in the treatment of cough and fever. University of KwaZulu- Natal Pietermaritzburg, South Africa.

Integrate

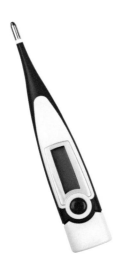 Nothing will make a parent more nervous than a child with a fever. Though conventional wisdom tells us there is nothing to worry about, no one wants their child to suffer. Use the easy guide to fever and other symptom relief in our 90-Day Plan Cheat Sheet in the section on Colds. From fever to coughs, this brochure will be your go-to guide for helping your children feel better fast.

Did you know?

A fever can be a good indication that an infection may be present. Drugs stop the fever immediately but also stop the body's "alert system." The application of essential oils can help the body to fight infections, viruses, and other germs with the fever. A low fever can show that the body is trying to do the right thing. Most bacteria and viruses like to live at body temperature; so if the temperature is raised, "bugs" are killed off. Research shows that our fears that fever is harmful originated after the introduction of over-the-counter fever-reducing drugs like Tylenol and Advil.

Dive In!

Growing Up Green: Baby and Child Care: Volume 2 in the Bestselling Green This! Series by Deirdre Imus (Paperback, 2008).

The Baby Book, Revised Edition: Everything You Need to Know About Your Baby from Birth to Age Two by William Sears, Martha Sears, Robert Sears, and James Sears (Paperback 2013).

Cheat Sheet

MONTH 1
GI Cleansing Formula
lavender
Daily Supplements Pack
Probiotic Defense Formula

MONTH 2
Daily Supplements Pack
peppermint
Probiotic Defense Formula

MONTH 3
lemon
Probiotic Defense Formula
Daily Supplements Pack
Calming Blend

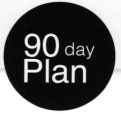

90 day Plan

Focus

In a world constantly pulling us in hundreds of directions, focus is a daily challenge. Calming the nervous system and quieting the mind is key.

Our Approach

APPLY *frankincense*, *rosemary*, and *Grounding Blend* to the temples and to the back of the neck and *Focus Blend* to the temples and the big toes.

TRY *Daily Supplements Pack* capsules or *Omega-3 Fish Oil* and *Chewable Multivitamins* twice a day to feed your brain with good nutrition to keep your mind focused. Boost it with *Energy & Stamina Complex*.

DIFFUSE *peppermint* when you need to concentrate, study, or work for long periods of time.

The mind works best in 20–30 minute increments. Give yourself a break, even for a minute or two while you are working on long-term projects. You will be amazed at how much more productive you become. A timer is a great tool.

Your Inner Geek

Rosemary has a long history as a memory enhancing herb—thousands of years ago the Greeks called it the herb of remembrance. Now doctors in Israel have completed trials using drugs containing rosemary oil. They discovered that many patients who have Alzheimer's disease have a shortage of a brain chemical called acetylcholine, which plays a key role in cognition and reasoning. Scientists found rosemary oil contains half a dozen compounds known to prevent the breakdown of acetylcholine. Students have also reported feeling livelier and more receptive to information after smelling the oil. *Daily Mail*, UK, April 2013

Multiple clinical trials have evaluated ginkgo for a syndrome called "cerebral insufficiency." This condition, more commonly diagnosed in Europe than in the United States, may include poor concentration, confusion, absentmindedness, decreased physical performance, fatigue, headache, dizziness, depression, and anxiety. It is believed that cerebral insufficiency is caused by decreased blood flow to the brain due to clogged blood vessels. Some research has reported benefits of ginkgo in patients with these symptoms, but most have been poorly designed and without reliable results.

Mayo Clinic

Integrate

Do you have a plan? It's hard to focus without one. We spend so much of our time worrying and wondering, which significantly cuts into our productivity. Whether using a 90-Day Plan for a health or business goal, you will find that setting goals in 90-day increments will significantly raise your productivity and help secure financial freedom.

Did you know?

Scientists have known for some time that the human brain's ability to stay calm and focused is limited and can be overwhelmed by the constant noise and hectic, jangling demands of city living, sometimes resulting in a condition informally known as brain fatigue. With brain fatigue, you are easily distracted, forgetful, and mentally flighty.

But an innovative new study from Scotland suggests that you can ease brain fatigue simply by strolling through a leafy park. The study, published in March 2013 in *The British Journal of Sports Medicine* by researchers at Heriot-Watt University in Edinburgh and the University of Edinburgh found that "Natural environments still engage" the brain, but the attention demanded "is effortless. It's called involuntary attention in psychology. It holds our attention while at the same time allowing scope for reflection," and providing a palliative to the nonstop attentional demands of typical city streets.

Dive In!

"It's a Smart, Smart, Smart World" by Nicholas Kristof, *The New York Times*, December 12, 2012.

Ogosport Mezo Disks: a floatable, portable, durable, and flexible game that helps relieve stress by bouncing balls up to 150 feet off mini trampolines. Ogosport Disk provides hours of adaptable entertainment for the whole family while boosting concentration and hand-eye coordination. Available at marblesthebrainstore.com

Play: How it Shapes the Brain, Opens the Imagination, and Invigorates the Soul by Stuart Brown and Christopher Vaughan (Paperback, 2010).

Cheat Sheet

MONTH 1
Focus Blend
Daily Supplements Pack
Energy & Stamina Complex

MONTH 2
Grounding Blend
Daily Supplements Pack
Energy & Stamina Complex

MONTH 3
rosemary
frankincense
Daily Supplements Pack
Energy & Stamina Complex

CHILDREN
Focus Blend
Chewable Multivitamin
Omega-3 Fish Oil
peppermint

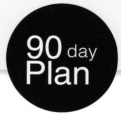

90 day Plan

From detoxification to metabolism, the liver and gallbladder play key roles in digestion, cleansing, and providing nourishment. If the liver is not functioning at a high level, nutrients will not be absorbed efficiently.

Our Approach

APPLY 2 drops of *cilantro, juniper,* and *Detoxification Blend* over the liver (across the abdomen) 2 times daily. Warm compresses may be added as well.

TRY the *Daily Supplements Pack* capsules and 2–4 drops of *cilantro* and *Invigorating Blend* in a capsule daily; add *Detoxification Complex* for further support.

DIFFUSE *Protective Blend* daily to keep your home and office environment clean. The liver serves as a filter for toxins, both airborne and ingested. The less the liver has to process, the healthier you will be.

Your Inner Geek

 Garlic contains numerous sulfur-containing compounds that activate the liver enzymes responsible for flushing out toxins from the body. This bulbous relative of the onion also contains allicin and selenium, two powerful nutrients proven to help protect the liver from toxic damage and aid it in the detoxification process. *Natural News*, May 2012

Multiple studies from Europe suggest benefits of oral milk thistle for cirrhosis. In experiments up to five years long, milk thistle has improved liver function and decreased the number of deaths that occur in cirrhotic patients. Mayo Clinic

Since most gallstones are composed of cholesterol, diet plays a role in their formation. Try this: Increase fiber and vitamin C, drink more water, lose weight slowly, and limit your sugar intake.

Integrate

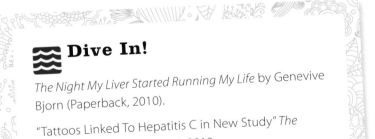 Essential oils are amazing detoxifiers. Whether applied, diffused, or ingested, these mighty oils are capable of eliminating the bad and avoiding the good. Share these wonderful detoxifiers with your friends and family. Their livers will thank you for it!

Did you know?

Although the liver can be partially removed and the gallbladder removed completely due to serious illness, keeping them healthy and strong should be paramount and surgery avoided whenever possible.

Most toxins or poisons reach our bloodstream when we swallow or inhale them. Others pass through the skin; while still others are released by dying cells or invading bacteria. Many of these toxins pass through the liver—the body's waste-purification plant—where they are broken down and removed from the blood before they can do their dirty work. Laurie Barclay, MD.

Dive In!

The Night My Liver Started Running My Life by Genevive Bjorn (Paperback, 2010).

"Tattoos Linked To Hepatitis C in New Study" *The Huffington Post*, January 24, 2013.

Cheat Sheet

MONTH 1
Daily Supplements Pack
Detoxification Blend
Detoxification Complex

MONTH 2
cilantro
Juniper
Daily Supplements Pack
Detoxification Complex

MONTH 3
Invigorating Blend
Daily Supplements Pack
Detoxification Complex

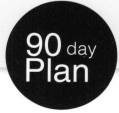

90 day **Plan**

Hair Care

Some of the most toxic products on the market today are found in haircare products. Because we wash our hair often and sometimes apply many products to our hair and scalp, we are putting our health at risk if we are not aware of the ingredients that we are using on our heads.

Our Approach

TRY the *Daily Supplements Pack* twice a day. Feeding your body well will also yield strong, beautiful hair.

APPLY essential oil–infused *Protecting Shampoo* and *Smoothing Conditioner*. For easy styling, apply essential oil–infused *Hair Glaze* to damp hair. To protect and repair scalp and dry ends, use a essential oil *Hair Serum* before and/or after blow drying.

> Try this to avoid lice: In a 4 ounce bottle filled with water, add 3 drops each of *rosemary*, *orange,* and *peppermint*. Shake well each time before using. Spray on hair daily before going out. It can also be sprayed on clothes, coats, bedding, and plush toys.

Your Inner Geek

Orange essential oil works from within, and this is one reason it is used in aromatherapies. Its fragrance has a soothing effect on the mind and can bust stress. Therefore, using orange oil on the hair has stabilizing effects on the nervous system, which in turn brings out calming effects on the mind, the body, and all the other organs. Thus, the scalp also receives an enriched supply of blood, with optimum usage made of the nutrients.

Another vital benefit of orange oil for hair care is its pest-exterminating properties. For lice-ridden hair, haircare treatments with orange oil are extremely beneficial because of their scalp-cleansing properties. *ifood.TV*

Integrate

The change of seasons and outdoor activities can be especially damaging and stressful to the hair. From swimming to sun stress, your hair certainly takes a beating in the summer. Avoid harmful ingredients such as sodium laurel sulfate and any type of paraben. Visit our social media sites for other great haircare and beauty tips.

Did you know?

Gentle cleansing agents derived from sources like coconut, nuts, and palm oil bring foam, spreadability, and a deeper clean into the shower. (Coconut derivatives are the most popular cleansers. On labels seek out words that begin with "coco" or "cocyl" in the ingredients list.) When you lather up with a natural shampoo, add water to generate extra foam instead of slopping on more product. Because they're made with oils, adding more shampoo adds more oil to the scalp, leaving hair limp.

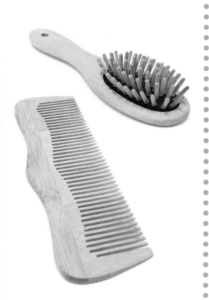

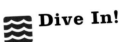 **Dive In!**

"Are You Having an Old Hair Day? Latest Anti-Aging Product Push is Pricey Hair Care; Way Beyond Gray" by Elizabeth Holmes, *Wall Street Journal*, April 4, 2013.

Organic Body Care Recipes: 175 Homemade Herbal Formulas for Glowing Skin & a Vibrant Self by Stephanie Tourles (Paperback, 2007).

Cheat Sheet

MONTH 1
Hair Glaze
Daily Supplements Pack
Protecting Shampoo
Smoothing Conditioner

MONTH 2
Daily Supplements Pack
Protecting Shampoo
Smoothing Conditioner
Hair Serum

MONTH 3
Daily Supplements Pack
Hair Glaze
Protecting Shampoo
Smoothing Conditioner

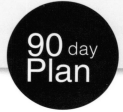

90 day **Plan**

Headaches

From a dull nagging pain to debilitating migraines, headaches are very common. Knowing the source of your headache will help you use your essential oils more effectively. Treatment for a sinus headache may differ from one caused by stress or hormone imbalance.

Our Approach

APPLY *Soothing Blend* and *Tension Blend* to the temples, forehead, and the back of the neck.

TRY the *Daily Supplements Pack* twice daily to lay a good nutritional foundation.

DIFFUSE *peppermint* or *basil* during your headache. Take 15 minutes to lie down and breathe.

Science suggests that you can help prevent the onset of migraines by providing sufficient nutrients to your body that help prevent blood vessel constriction. Try foods like flax seeds or fish for omega-3 and millet or spinach for B vitamins and magnesium.

Your Inner Geek

 Basil can be used to treat digestive problems, poor circulation, kidney ailments, headaches, and inflammation. In addition, recent studies have shown that basil's water-soluble flavonoids (orientin and vicenin) can prevent free-radical damage in cells, helping reduce cancer risk. Cheryl Meyers, *Alternative Medicine*

"The medicinal use of peppermint and other mint plants probably dates back to the herbal pharmacopoeia of ancient Greece, where peppermint leaf traditionally was used internally as a digestive aid and for management of gallbladder disease; it also was inhaled for upper respiratory symptoms and cough," writes Benjamin Kligler, MD, Albert Einstein College of Medicine, Yeshiva University, New York, and Sapna Chaudhary, DO, Beth

Cheat Sheet

Israel Continuum Center for Health and Healing, New York.

"Peppermint oil, which is extracted from the stem, leaves, and flowers of the plant, has become popular as a treatment for a variety of conditions, including irritable bowel syndrome (IBS), headache, and non-ulcer dyspepsia."
Medscape

Integrate

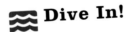 Headaches have many root causes and are often difficult to diagnose. No matter what the cause of the pain, essential oils can have a positive effect on eliminating and preventing pain. Our basic pain relief program in the 90-Day Plan Cheat Sheet in the section on Pain Relief can help to adjust your body's natural ability to reduce inflammation and minimize headaches.

Did you know?

Over 150 studies have looked into the connection between food allergies and migraines. Some of the top migraine-inducing foods identified include wheat, cow's milk, grain cereals, sugar, yeast, corn, citrus, and eggs.

≋ Dive In!

"Why That Banana or Onion Might Feel like Three Martinis" by Sumathi Reddy *Wall Street Journal*, December 18, 2012.

"How Diet and Supplements Can Help Prevent Migraines," by Dr. Joseph Mercola, *mercola.com*, December 24, 2012.

MONTH 1
Daily Supplements Pack
Tension Blend

MONTH 2
Soothing Blend
Daily Supplements Pack

MONTH 3
basil
peppermint
Daily Supplements Pack

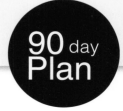

90 day Plan

Heart Health

The heart is considered the "center" of our emotions, but it is also vital to our overall health and longevity. Taking care of your heart means eating well, getting plenty of rest, and exercising daily.

Our Approach

APPLY *Calming Blend*, *cypress*, *helichrysum*, *juniper,* and *ylang ylang* over the heart 1–2 times daily if you are dealing with a cardiovascular problem or a chronic condition. To support your heart on a regular basis, repeat 1–2 times a week.

TRY the *Daily Supplements Pack* twice daily. We also like taking *Digestive Enzyme Complex* in addition to the above supplements for extra support.

DIFFUSE *Calming Blend* to reduce stress.

Good circulation will put less stress on the heart. Try massaging your legs and arms with cypress oil to promote good circulation; give extra attention to the hands and feet.

Your Inner Geek

Because stress can be a significant contributor to heart disease, it is important to find ways to alleviate it, says Lori Mosca, MD, director of preventive cardiology at New York-Presbyterian Hospital. Taking time to decompress in a quiet place works wonders. Mosca advises her patients to slip into something comfortable, like a warm, scent-filled bath. The combination of pleasant aroma and a relaxing read will put you in a peaceful mood. In her book, *Heart to Heart*, Mosca recommends experimenting with fragrant oils, including lavender, sandalwood, and ylang ylang, until you find the one that provides the benefit you are seeking.

Integrate

Coronary heart disease, high blood pressure, stroke, heart attacks, and angina can all be brought on by the disruption of hormone balance caused by synthetic hormones found in foods, medicines, birth control, or personal care products. Balancing your hormones naturally can help support a healthy heart. Women, follow our tips in the 90-Day Plan Cheat Sheet in the section on Women's Health.

Did you know?

The Weston Price Foundation states, "Mental and physical stress, with its related continuous flow of adrenaline, uses up magnesium rapidly, as adrenaline affects heart rate, blood pressure, vascular constriction and muscle contraction—actions that all demand steady supplies of magnesium for smooth function."

An easy way to get more magnesium is by eating organic green, leafy vegetables. Other foods high in magnesium include rice, wheat or oat bran, spinach, artichokes, dried herbs, squash pumpkin and watermelon seeds, dark chocolate cocoa powder, flax and sesame seeds, Brazil nuts, sunflower seeds, almonds, and pine nuts.

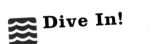 **Dive In!**

"What Causes Heart Disease?" by Sally Fallon and Mary G. Enig, PhD, westonprice.org, March 1, 2001.

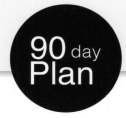

Cheat Sheet

MONTH 1
juniper
Daily Supplements Pack
Calming Blend
Digestive Enzyme
Complex

MONTH 2
cypress
Daily Supplements Pack
Digestive Enzyme
Complex
ylang ylang

MONTH 3
helichrysum
Daily Supplements Pack
Digestive Enzyme
Complex

90 day **Plan**

Immune Support

Your best defense against any illness is a strong immune system. The immune system is constantly changing, trying to stay ahead of everything that attacks our bodies. Providing support to this system should be a daily pursuit.

Our Approach

APPLY 1–2 drops of **Protective Blend** to the bottoms of the feet once or twice a day during the fall and winter months. In the spring and summer, apply 1–2 drops of **Cleansing Blend** to the bottoms of the feet once or twice a day,

TRY taking a **Protective Softgel** during the day and a **Probiotic Defense Formula** capsule at night before bed (continue using daily to help strengthen immunity). When illness does strike, add **Essential Oil Cellular Complex**.

DIFFUSE **Protective Blend** and **Cleansing Blend**.

Vitamin C tops the list of immune boosters for many reasons. There has been more research about the immune-boosting effects of vitamin C than perhaps any other nutrient.
Dr. William Sears

Your Inner Geek

 "Probiotics, microorganisms that have a favorable influence on… the host by their effect on the intestinal flora, may play a role in improving human health." Kent L. Erickson and Neil E. Hubbard, American Society for Nutritional Sciences, 2000.

A 1990 study showed that people who take aspirin and Tylenol (acetaminophen) suppress their body's ability to produce antibodies that destroy the cold virus, thus causing the body to take longer to fight the cold and accounting for any secondary infections and post-nasal drip (J Infect Dis, Dec 1990; 162(6):1277-82).

Researchers have found that some essential oils—oregano, thyme, and rosewood oils, in particular—create an autolytic (destruction of cells and tissues by enzymes produced by the cells themselves) reaction in organisms, including streptococcus

pneumonia.
Dr. Diane Horne of Weber State University, Ogden, Utah, *Natural News*.

Integrate

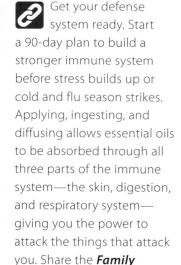

Get your defense system ready. Start a 90-day plan to build a stronger immune system before stress builds up or cold and flu season strikes. Applying, ingesting, and diffusing allows essential oils to be absorbed through all three parts of the immune system—the skin, digestion, and respiratory system—giving you the power to attack the things that attack you. Share the **Family Healthcare Kit** with friends to help them stay healthy too!

Did you know?

The greatest advantage an essential oil has over something that is man-made is its ability to quickly adapt to its surroundings. Just like a bacteria can turn into a "super bug," an essential oil can adapt to the germ it's fighting. Vaccines, antibiotics, and other medicines cannot adapt or change to fit a situation. If the germ gets ahead of your medicine, the germ will win every time. On the other hand, medicinal plants keep coming back stronger and smarter.

≋ Dive In!

"Antimicrobial Resistance in the European Union and the World" by Dr. Margaret Chan, Director-General of the World Health Organization, March 14, 2012. The EU's contributions to the solutions of the global antimicrobial resistance problem. Keynote address at the conference on Combating Antimicrobial Resistance: Time for Joint Action.

Super Immunity: The Essential Nutrition Guide for Boosting Your Body's Defenses to Live Longer, Stronger, and Disease Free by Joel Fuhrman (Hardcover, 2011).

Cheat Sheet

MONTH 1
Protective Blend
Essential Oil Cellular Complex
Protective Softgels
Probiotic Defense Formula

MONTH 2
Cleansing Blend
Essential Oil Cellular Complex
Protective Softgels
Probiotic Defense Formula

MONTH 3
Protective Blend
Essential Oil Cellular Complex
Protective Softgels
Probiotic Defense Formula

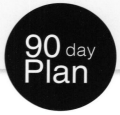

90 day **Plan**

Kidney / Bladder

The kidneys produce urine, which contains the byproducts of metabolism—salts, toxins, and water. Urine is then eliminated through the bladder. These two organs get rid of waste that would end up in the blood.

Our Approach

APPLY 1–2 drops of *juniper* or ***Detoxification Blend*** to the lower back.

TRY ***Detoxification Complex*** and the ***Daily Supplements Pack***. Always drink plenty of water.

DIFFUSE ***Protective Blend*** into the air to reduce stress on the body.

Lemongrass and ***rosemary*** are natural diuretics. If you find that you need to reduce fluid in your body, try these natural solutions, and drink plenty of water. The minerals in the water keep the body from becoming too dehydrated.

Your Inner Geek

 Dandelion root (found in ***Detoxification Complex***) has a long history of supporting kidney health and has been employed as a diuretic for over 2000 years in both Traditional Chinese and Ayurvedic medicine. This historical data suggests that various species of dandelion have been widely used for urinary and renal diseases and to enhance the elimination of fluids. "The Diuretic Effect in Human Subjects of an Extract of *Taraxacum officinale* Folium over a Single Day," *Journal of Alternative and Complementary Medicine*, August 2009.

Also contained in ***Detoxification Complex*** is burdock root. Burdock may be nature's best blood purifier and "alterative," which has numerous beneficial effects on the body. Burdock appears to stimulate the efficient removal of waste products and is said to cleanse and eliminate long-term impurities from the blood through its action on both the

> **But I know all about love already. I know precious little about kidneys.**
> —Aldous Huxley

liver and kidneys. The increased flow of urine relieves both the kidney and lymphatic system with many beneficial effects. *Organic Herbs Medicine Cabinet*

Integrate

Women often suffer from kidney and bladder infections. Supporting the kidneys in puberty can help a young woman strengthen her kidneys and bladder to prevent infections from occurring. Getting your hormones working properly goes a long way in supporting other systems of the body too. Try our 90-Day Plan Cheat Sheet in the Women's Health section to put your body on the right track. Men who struggle with prostate issues may also face an over active bladder. Use our tips in this section to help reduce symptoms.

Did you know?

The National Association For Continence (NAFC) reports that about 25 million adult Americans experience transient or chronic problems with urinary incontinence—and the vast majority who struggle with passing urine accidentally, around 75 percent, are women.

According to the Mayo Clinic website, the major types of medications used to relieve urinary incontinence are anticholinergics, alpha-adrenergic agonists, and estrogen. All these drugs are laden with potential side effects, ranging from dry mouth, dizziness, constipation, heartburn, blurry vision, and urinary retention to impaired memory, confusion, and even cancer.

Supplements help to rest the kidneys, allowing them to recover, repair, and function optimally once more. A delicate balance of diet, fluids, supplements, and exercise is needed to repair the kidneys and provide the rest they need for a long and healthy future. Natural News, February 2009.

Dive In!

"The Claim: Too Much Cola Can Cause Kidney Problems" by Anahad O'Connor, The New York Times, January 22, 2008.

"Bladder Cancer a Growing Concern for Smokers" by Anahad O'Connor, The New York Times, August 17, 2011.

Cheat Sheet

MONTH 1
Protective Blend
Daily Supplements Pack
Detoxification Complex

MONTH 2
Protective Blend
Daily Supplements Pack
Detoxification Complex

MONTH 3
Protective Blend
Daily Supplements Pack
Detoxification Complex

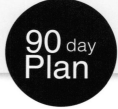

90 day Plan

Libido

Our libido is a combination of the mind and body. Sex drive can be effected by many factors, including hormones, family, work, age, medications, stress, and more.

Our Approach

APPLY 1 drop of **sandalwood**, **rose,** or **ylang ylang** on you or your partner; dilute generously with **coconut oil** on sensitive areas or for a full body massage.

TRY using the **Daily Supplements Pack** and the **Energy & Stamina Complex** as directed daily.

DIFFUSE the **Women's Blend** to set the mood.

Enjoying an active sex life is essential to our well-being, and the foods we eat play a large role in ensuring that we feel sexy. Some of the foods that help turn us on include pumpkin seeds, avocados, bee pollen, and figs. Supplements containing vitamin E and omega-3 fatty acids can also help. **Ginger** has been used for centuries as a highly effective aid to digestion, but its classification as a natural aphrodisiac comes from its ability to increase circulation.

Your Inner Geek

According to a May 2008 report, "Sexual desire, as well as orgasm, are controlled by various influences on the brain and nervous system. Brain imaging studies show that achieving orgasm involves far more than arousal. It requires a release of inhibitions, culminating in a shutdown of the brain's center of vigilance in both sexes, and widespread neural power failure in women. Without that initial psychological impetus, potency pills have no effect." *Scientific American*

The ability of aroma to enhance libido and sexual arousal has been explored and documented by Dr. Alan Hirsch, Director of Chicago's Smell & Taste Treatment and Research Center, with lavender having the greatest effect.

> **Sex appeal is fifty percent what you've got and fifty percent what people think you've got.—Sophia Loren**

Integrate

Balancing your hormones is key to a healthy libido. Whether you are young or old, supporting your hormones is necessary. Your libido can change over time with fluctuating hormones. If you are not feeling the way you would like, get a blood test done to have your hormones checked. If you choose to try something natural, start with stress-reducing oil blends like **Calming Blend** (men and women), **Grounding Blend**, and **Women's Monthly Blend** (women).

Did you know?

Essential oils can be very effective in stimulating the libido. **Sandalwood** has been known since ancient times to improve blood flow, balance mood, and stimulate interest. Because its scent is close to a man's, it is especially effective for women. **Jasmine** is known to tame anger, raise interest, and inspire passion. **Ylang ylang**, jasmine's close counterpart, is less expensive and has similar properties. **Rose**, perhaps the most expensive and rare essential oil, is also one of the most effective. From Cleopatra to Snow White, rose has been associated with love, passion, and romance. These oils can be applied neat to the pulse points or added to **coconut oil** to make a massage oil for you or your partner. While expensive, a small amount diffused in a closed room can also set a romantic mood.

≋ Dive In!

"7 Foods for Better Sex" by Joseph Mercola MD, Mercola.com, March 4, 2011.

Harvard Medical School, Sexuality in Midlife and Beyond by Jan Leslie MD and Suki Hanfling (Paperback, 2010).

Cheat Sheet

MONTH 1
coconut oil
Daily Supplements Pack
Energy & Stamina Complex
ylang ylang

MONTH 2
Daily Supplements Pack
Energy & Stamina Complex
sandalwood

MONTH 3
Daily Supplements Pack
Energy & Stamina Complex
Women's Blend

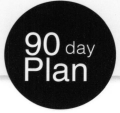

90 day **Plan**

Men's Health

Beginning a regimen of supplements, whole foods, and essential oils may protect you from ailments that are common to men. Making small changes at any age can have a great effect on your health, longevity, and strength. You are your own best caretaker.

Our Approach

APPLY *Joyful Blend* or *Grounding Blend* daily instead of chemically-based colognes and aftershave products.

TRY using the *Daily Supplements Pack* and *Energy & Stamina Complex* daily. These supplements help to strengthen bones, ligaments, and muscles and increase energy, reduce stress, and provide nutritional balance. Use a *Protective Beadlet* for fresh breath and immune support.

DIFFUSE *Calming Blend* to reduce stress and *Joyful Blend* or *peppermint* to increase productivity at home or at the office.

In studies on lab animals, the omega-3 fatty acids EPA & DHA in fish oil inhibited tumors. Harvard researchers also found that men who ate fish 3 times a week reduced their risk of aggressive prostate cancer by 25%—*Omega-3 Fish Oil* contains 1000 mg of fish oil concentrate—including both EPA and DHA.

Your Inner Geek

 The supplement coenzyme Q10, found in *Cellular Vitality Complex* and *Energy & Stamina Complex*, is thought to improve heart function. In a double-blind trial, 145 people who had recently experienced a heart attack were given either a placebo or 120 mg of CoQ10 daily for 28 days. The results showed that participants receiving CoQ10 experienced significantly fewer heart-related problems, such as episodes of angina, arrhythmia, or recurrent heart attacks. CoQ10 taken in combination with the mineral selenium has also shown promise for people who have survived a heart attack (NYU Langone Medical Center).

"Boswellic acids interact with several different proteins that are part of inflammatory reactions," says Prof. Dr. Oliver Werz of Friedrich Schiller Jena University, Germany. "Boswellic acids block [certain] enzymes efficiently and thereby reduce the inflammatory reaction."

Boswellic acids also have fewer side effects than today's prevalent anti-inflammatory treatments.

Integrate

Don't feel overwhelmed by the thought of adding a healthy regimen to your life. Simple, economical steps can be easily taken following the 90-Day Plan. Learning how to use natural products is as easy as 1-2-3—apply, diffuse, ingest.

Did you know?

Men often feel like they have to hold up the world, allowing the stress of family and work to come before their health, until a crisis occurs.

Here are some of the active ingredients in the natural supplements listed in the **Our Approach** section: calcium & vitamin D, to help you maintain a healthy weight and strengthen bones; chromium, to help ward off diabetes; boswellic acid, to grease your joints; folate, to fight against Alzheimer's and Parkinson's diseases; omega-3, to protect your heart; selenium, to fight cancer; and vitamin E, to slow aging.

Dive In!

"Like Charlemagne, You've Got Gout," *The New York Times*, June 20, 2005.

"It's No Contact Sport, but Golf Can Leave a Duffer Banged Up," The New York Times, June 20, 2005.

Cheat Sheet

MONTH 1
Grounding Blend
Daily Supplements Pack
Energy & Stamina Complex
Protective Beadlets

MONTH 2
Grounding Blend
Daily Supplements Pack
Energy & Stamina Complex
Protective Beadlets

MONTH 3
Daily Supplements Pack
Energy & Stamina Complex
peppermint
Calming Blend

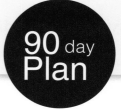

90 day Plan

Nausea, Vomiting, Upset Stomach

Nausea, vomiting, or upset stomach is our body's way of ridding itself of toxins. When we digest food, our immune system slows down. Not eating heavily allows the immune system to kick into gear. So listen to your body when symptoms strike.

Our Approach

APPLY *ginger*, *peppermint,* or *Digestive Blend* to the abdomen, back, and feet.

TRY *ginger*, *peppermint,* or *Digestive Blend* in a glass of water or a drop or two in a capsule, or take *Detoxification Complex*. Sip the water with oils slowly. Drinking too much water can encourage vomiting. Once the nausea has subsided, fortify the gut with *Probiotic Defense Formula*.

DIFFUSE or inhale *ginger, peppermint,* or *Digestive Blend*.

Essential oils can be put in a cup of warm water and consumed like tea or put into a warm bath. But remember, if it's too hot for you to drink or bathe in, then it's too hot for the oil. Heating oils at extremely high temperatures may damage the oil. Warm water is also easier for the body to assimilate.

Your Inner Geek

In the largest study to date evaluating the benefits of ginger for patients undergoing chemotherapy, as little as one-quarter of a teaspoon of ginger cut symptoms of nausea by 40% (University of Rochester).

Preliminary studies suggest that direct contact with *peppermint* oil may be helpful in reducing spasms in the esophagus and intestines during endoscopies and other medical procedures. There is some evidence that enteric-coated peppermint oil (supplements that are coated so that they are not absorbed by the body until they reach the small intestine) might be helpful in treating symptoms of irritable bowel syndrome, such as cramps (American Cancer Society).

> By swallowing evil words unsaid, no one has ever harmed his stomach.
> —Winston Churchill

Integrate

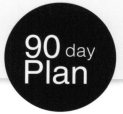 Nausea may be only one of the many symptoms you experience when ill. What can start off as an upset stomach can turn into fever, cough, runny nose, and more overnight. Look at the section on Immune Support for additional 90-Day Plan suggestions.

Did you know?

Can't stand to drink anything? Try making an ice cube with a drop of essential oil. A little goes a long way, so you may want to add a drop of **peppermint** to a pitcher of water (mix well with a whisk and pour immediately, as the oil tends to float to the top), and then fill your ice tray. This not only helps to flavor cool drinks but also sucking on an ice cube when you are sick may be easier to tolerate than a full glass of water.

The essential oil of **ginger** is a nausea relief must-have. **Ginger** is widely used for digestive issues of all types, as it improves digestion, calms nausea, encourages gastric juices to form, and has countless other digestive benefits. Through scent, essential oils can travel to the limbic system of your brain, which responds by releasing neurotransmitters and hormones to help calm your stomach. Essential oils also work when applied topically, as they travel through the skin into the blood stream..

≋ Dive In!

What to Expect, Eating Well When You're Expecting by Heidi Murkoff and Sharon Mazel (Paperback, 2005).

Animal, Vegetable, Miracle: A Year of Food Life by Barbara Kingsolver, Camille Kingsolver, and Steven L. Hopp (Paperback, 2008).

Treatment Alternatives for Children by Lawrence Rosen MD and Jeff Cohen with contributors Carrie Donegan and Elena Yordán (Paperback 2012).

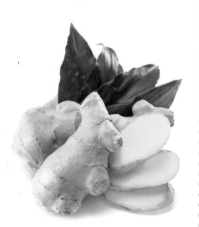

Cheat Sheet

MONTH 1
Digestive Blend
ginger
Probiotic Defense Formula
peppermint

MONTH 2
Digestive Softgels
Probiotic Defense Formula
peppermint

MONTH 3
Digestive Blend
ginger
Probiotic Defense Formula

90 day
Plan

Nutrition

Nothing is a better friend to nutrition than an essential oil. Combine an essential oil with a whole food or a whole food supplement, and you have a powerful health tool.

Our Approach

APPLY your favorite essential oils to the soles of your feet daily to help slowly correct imbalances in your body. We like *Protective Blend* and *Grounding Blend* for daily immune, hormone, and skeletal support. Essential oils have also been seen to help with the absorption of nutrients.

TRY the *Daily Supplements Pack* twice daily. For additional nutritional support, add *Digestive Enzyme Complex* and *Probiotic Defense Formula*.

DIFFUSE *lemon*, *Invigorating Blend,* or *Calming Blend*. Coniferous oils like *white fir* and *spruce* can also help oxygenate the blood, increasing nutritional absorption.

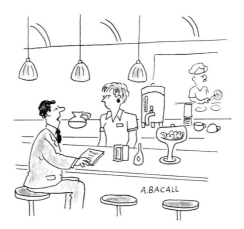

"Let me have 20% fat, 40% carbohydrate, 40% protein and a cup of tea."

Your Inner Geek

Astaxanthin (pronounced "asta-ZAN-thin" and found in *Vegan Essential Oil Omega Complex* and *Essential Oil Omega Complex*) is a naturally-occurring carotenoid and powerful antioxidant. Discussed at length by Dr. Mehmet Oz, Dr. Joseph Mercola, and others, here are the 5 major reasons you want to add this into your nutritional regimen every day:

- Astaxanthin can help relieve pain and inflammation—acting both as a potent pain reliever and blocker of inflammatory compounds that drive many chronic diseases.
- Astaxanthin helps fight fatigue and is indicated for recovery of muscles, better endurance, enhanced strength, and improved energy levels.
- Astaxanthin supports eye health, including helping diabetic retinopathy, macular degeneration, eye strain, and seeing in fine detail.

Have fun with your food—take it on the go! Making whole foods at home and carrying them in fun containers like a Bento box can help to break up the monotony. Treat yourself to new and different condiments like lemon wedges, wasabi, salsa, or citrus oils to make lunch a treat for all the senses.

- Astaxanthin cleans up the cells of the body with the ability to protect both the fat soluble and water soluble parts of the cell.
- Astaxanthin provides skin and sunscreen protection, improving skin moisture levels, smoothness, elasticity, fine wrinkles, spots, or freckles. —Huffington Post

Integrate

One way to increase your nutrition is to get rid of toxins that have built up in your fat. Essential oils and oil–enhanced supplements are very effective in burning fats and releasing toxins, with citrus oils having been know as fat burners for years. Learn easy tips on how to use these and other oils and supplements to get rid of toxins and increase nutrition on our social media sites.

Did you know?

The Standard American Diet known as "SAD" is unfortunately significantly lacking important nutrients. The key components in this diet—processed foods—are filled with preservatives, salt, and sugars (both refined and artificial), which can be addicting and contain empty calories. Getting on a whole-food supplementation program and a "clean eating" diet including a variety of vegetables and fruits is one way to break the cycle of food addiction and sluggish metabolism. Eating cleanly means you don't have to count calories. Clean foods like vegetables and fruits, nuts, seeds, lean meats, eggs, fish, and some whole grains have fewer calories than processed foods and are packed with nutrition. Watch portion sizes!

Essential oils added to foods can provide the added "oomph" or "umami" that make a dish delicious and stimulating to all the elements of taste: sweet, salty, bitter, and sour. Lastly, eating healthily can help to support healing and rebuild the spirit during times of stress..

Dive In!

"Breeding the Nutrition Out of Our Food" by Jo Robinson, *The New York Times--Sunday Review*, May 25, 2013.

Eating on the Wild Side: The Missing Link to Optimum Health by Jo Robinson (Hardcover 2013).

"Is Sugar Toxic?" by Gary Taubes, *The New York Times Sunday Magazine*, April 13, 2011).

Cheat Sheet

MONTH 1
Daily Supplements Pack
Protective Blend
Probiotic Defense Formula
Digestive Enzyme
Complex

MONTH 2
lemon
Grounding Blend
Daily Supplements Pack
Probiotic Defense Formula
Digestive Enzyme
Complex

MONTH 3
Invigorating Blend
Daily Supplements Pack
Probiotic Defense Formula
Calming Blend
Digestive Enzyme
Complex

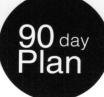
90 day **Plan**

Pain Relief

Pain can strike when we are not expecting it and can seem to last with no end in sight. Fighting the root cause of your pain is key to relieving it. Essential oils are effective because they go right to work at the cellular level.

Our Approach

APPLY *Soothing Blend* and *Tension Blend* to the area of pain. If you have nerve pain, add a *Soothing Rub* on top for added power. For a full-body massage, use the oils in the **Aroma Massage Kit**.

TRY the *Daily Supplements Pack* twice daily.

DIFFUSE *Calming Blend*, *lavender*, or another calming oil. Tension and stress can exacerbate pain. Relaxation can be the first step to pain relief.

Try different applications of essential oils to alleviate pain: in warm baths, with warm or cool compresses, or in full-body massage. Essential blends like **Soothing Blend** or **Grounding Blend** or single oils like **wintergreen** applied before, during, or after acupuncture, yoga, chiropractic adjustments, or physical therapy can enhance the effects of these modalities.

Your Inner Geek

Camphor (found in *Soothing Rub*) has a long history of reducing pain. However, the mechanisms by which camphor works to ease irritation and pain are not entirely understood. It appears that camphor molecules penetrate the skin and combat the naturally produced chemicals that cause inflammation. Itchy skin, tight muscles, and swollen joints tend to subside fairly quickly after application. Camphor may also act as an anesthetic on nerves near the skin, further reducing painful symptoms related to arthritis or injury (WiseGEEK.com).

For pain, Dr. Mehmet Oz recommends *helichrysum* oil as an "alternative to over-the-counter pain medications. Derived from strawflower, this ancient remedy has been used for hundreds of years in Africa. Its powerful anti-inflammatory properties are excellent at reducing muscle tension and anxiety. In addition, helichrysum is very effective when used in the treatment of wounds, bug bites, burns, joint pain and arthritis."

Integrate

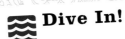 The 90-Day Plan Cheat Sheet for pain takes a two-pronged approach: oils and supplements. We find that using the two in combination is the winning formula. Pain is best defeated when attacked both from the inside and outside. Make a commitment, and be consistent. Keep up with the program for at least 90 days to get the results you desire.

Did you know?

You are never too old to relieve pain! Our friend Clara O. from New York writes: "I am an 80+ year old woman and have suffered pain in my joints for almost 40 years. Although I tried several drugs, the side effects were terrible. Now I use essential oils on my knees, shoulders, and feet — where I feel pain — both morning and night. While I have been using cypress and wintergreen for several years now, I recently added **Soothing Rub** with great success. I recommend it to all my friends."

Dive In!

"Optical Illusion Relieves Arthritis Pain: Arthritis Pain Is Reduced by Mirror Reflections of Healthier Joints" by Stephani Sutherland, *Scientific American*, May 23, 2012.

"Profiting From Pain: The Use of Narcotic Painkillers, or Opioids, Has Boomed Over the Past Decade as Drug Makers and Doctors Have Promoted Them" by Barry Meier, *The New York Times*, June 22, 2013.

Cheat Sheet

MONTH 1
Soothing Blend
Soothing Rub
Daily Supplements Pack
Tension Blend

MONTH 2
Aroma Massage Kit
Daily Supplements Pack
Calming Blend

MONTH 3
Soothing Blend
Soothing Rub
lavender
Daily Supplements Pack

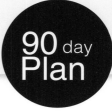

90 day **Plan**

Pregnancy

Using essential oils and supplements while pregnant or becoming pregnant is a personal choice that must be made with your spouse or partner and medical advisor.

Our Approach

APPLY the oil of your choice diluted with **coconut oil**. Even if you are used to using an oil neat, your skin sensitivity can change during pregnancy, and it's always best to be cautious. **Lemon**, **lavender**, **myrrh**, **vetiver,** and **ylang ylang** are traditional favorites of moms-to-be.

TRY a natural personal care product line of dental, hair, and skin care that can help limit your exposure to toxins. Be sure to take the prenatal vitamins your doctor recommends.

DIFFUSE or inhale **ginger**, **peppermint,** or **Digestive Blend** to limit nausea.

Your Inner Geek

 Fennel's use in promoting breast milk production dates back to ancient Greece, according to herbs2000.com, which states that the herb actively aids in breast milk secretion. Although there is no scientific evidence on the effectiveness of fennel seed for increasing milk production, according to breastfeeding.com, fennel in moderate amounts is safe for breastfeeding moms. As another possible benefit, *Alive Magazine* and herbs2000.com suggest that fennel may help alleviate digestive troubles for a nursing baby.

Ashley Turner of MindBodyGreen says, "Stretch marks appear when skin is overworked, which results in a weakening or breakdown of deep fibers." Stretch marks generally fade from red to silvery as weight decreases and skin returns to normal. When used as a preventative measure, **lavender** and **myrrh** help improve the elasticity of the skin, which can help decrease the amount of deep fiber damage and reduce the visible appearance of stretch marks. Either oil can be mixed with a carrier oil and be applied directly to the skin. Apply a small amount daily, and gently massage it into the hips, stomach, thighs, and any area that feels particularly taut, or on scar tissue. Pregnancy and the changes that occur afterward can be hard on your body and your hormones. **Vetiver** oil is known for being psychologically grounding, calming, and stabilizing, while **lemon** is known for its strong, purifying scent that revitalizes and uplifts. Either oil can be inhaled directly from the bottle or diffused in a room. Mild oils like lavender can be diffused in a baby's room. Use a water bowl with drop or two of essential oils for infants between six months and one year.

> ## A baby is a little bit of heaven on earth.
> ### —Unknown

Integrate

 Learning how to use essential oils safely and in multiple arenas can become a useful life tool. Limiting the number of chemicals in personal care, medications, and cleaners will help to green your body, environment, and your family. Follow the suggestions in the 90-Day Plan Cheat Sheet in the Cleaning section, for tips on how to make your home safe, natural, and clean for you and your baby.

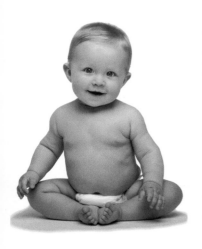

Did you know?

Nerve cells or neurons are produced in the fetus at an average rate of 250,000 per minute. But every human spent an hour as a single cell. Once you have seen a fetal heart beat, the risk of miscarriage lowers to 5%. Unborn babies can feel, see, and hear, so spend time stroking your belly and talking to your baby in the womb (welcomebabyhome.com).

Dive In!

"Should Doctors Warn Pregnant Women about Environmental Risks?: Most Doctors Do Not Warn Pregnant Patients about Chemicals, Pesticides or Even Mercury Contamination" by Jane Kay, Environmental Health News, Scientific American, December 10, 2012.

Do women eat more when expecting a boy? In 2003 a team of researchers from the U.S. and Europe studied the diets of 244 pregnant women during their second trimester and found that those carrying male fetuses ate, on average, 190 more calories per day than those carrying females. Those extra calories apparently made a beeline for the fetus, because the boy babies were heavier and their mothers did not pack on any more pounds than those carrying girls. "We found that birth weight of boys was on the average higher than that of girls," says senior author Dimitrios Trichopoulos, an epidemiologist at the Harvard School of Public Health in Boston. "Our interpretation is that boys are somehow programmed to be heavier than girls, and this requires higher caloric intake from the mother," he adds, speculating that testosterone from the fetal testicles might be involved in increasing the maternal appetite.

Cheat Sheet

MONTH 1
coconut oil
ginger
Daily Supplements Pack
ylang ylang

MONTH 2
lemon
Daily Supplements Pack
myrrh
peppermint

MONTH 3
lavender
Daily Supplements Pack
ylang ylang
vetiver

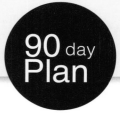

90 day
Plan

Skincare

The skin is the largest organ of the body. As part of the immune system, it protects us from outside invaders, helps to regulate body temperature, and reflects our age and state of health. Take care of your skin, and your skin will take care of you.

Our Approach

APPLY (for dry to normal skin) *Facial Cleanser* and then *Skin Toner*. Follow with *Anti-Aging Blend* and *Anti-Aging Moisturizer*. For additional moisturizing or for nighttime renewal, apply *Hydrating Cream*.

For oily skin, cleanse with *Face Wash* and then apply *Skin Toner*. Use *Topical Blend* on blemishes and trouble spots, and follow with *Skin Serum*. Two to three times a week, use *Invigorating Scrub* to help exfoliate. For your body, choose "clean" bath gels, soaps, and lotions, avoiding the ingredients in the Dive In! section. Our favorite spa products are the *Invigorating Bath Bar*, unscented *Hand & Body Lotion*, and *Rose Oil Hand Lotion*. Mix your favorite essential oil with *Hand & Body Lotion* to create your own lotion scents every day!

TRY the *Daily Supplements Pack* capsules twice daily.

DIFFUSE *Protective Blend* and *Cleansing Blend* daily to kill airborne toxins that can affect the skin.

Your Inner Geek

"Up until now, science was much more focused on finding the synthetic substitutes in beauty," says Shirin Valipour, a 24-year veteran of the beauty industry who started Orico, an organic skincare brand based in London. "Now there are labs around the world that are testing bioactive and natural ingredients and those clinically proven naturals are then becoming more available."
The New York Times

According to Patricia Davis in *Aromatherapy: An A-Z*, "Geranium oil is an astringent, antiseptic, and stimulant." Combine *geranium* oil with *rose* or *lavender* for greater effect.

Wash off your makeup at night!
Makeup contains harmful chemicals and will hold air pollutants to the skin, causing pores to become clogged and damaging the skin's surface. A clean face gives the body time to repair the skin while you sleep. During the day, try to resist touching your face. Our hands carry additional bacteria and harmful chemicals, including BPA, from receipts, money, and plastic water bottles that can aggravate a skin condition or cause allergies and breakouts.

Integrate

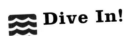

Many people battle skin allergies. From eczema to psoriasis, these irritating and often painful conditions can attack children and adults alike. Following our guide in the 90-Day Plan in the section on Allergies will put you on a 90-day path to better skin. Don't give up. It takes time for the skin to heal. Be patient knowing that your skin is being supported with the right oils and supplements.

NONE OF THE BAD—INGREDIENT PHILOSOPHY
When formulating skincare products, you should NEVER use the following:

- Artificial colors
- Diethanolamine (DEA)
- Formaldehyde donors
- Parabens
- Phthalates
- Propylene glycol
- Sodium laureth sulfate (SLES)
- Sodium lauryl sulfate (SLS)
- Toluene
- Triethanolamine (TEA)
- Animal testing

Did you know?

Face masks have been used since the time of Cleopatra. You can brighten your skin by combining a few simple ingredients. For dry skin, mix equal parts unripened papaya, plain whole milk, yogurt, and a few drops of **geranium** oil. For oily skin, mix equal parts avocado, cucumber, mineral rich green clay, and a few drops of **lemon** oil. Apply either as a mask to the skin, and allow to dry for 20 minutes. Rinse off with cool water, and pat dry (WholeLiving.com).

Dive In!

In her book, *Gorgeously Green*, Sophie Ulliano recommends avoiding these ingredients in your skin care products: Parabens (methyl-, ethyl-, propyl-, butyl-, and isobutyl-), Fragrance, Sodium Laurel Sulfate (SLS), and Talc.

Cheat Sheet

MONTH 1
Pick according to skin type:
Facial Cleanser
Skin Toner
Anti-Aging Moisturizer
Anti-Aging Blend
Daily Supplements Pack

MONTH 2
Invigorating Bath Bar
Rose Oil Hand Lotion
lavender
Daily Supplements Pack
Protective Blend

MONTH 3
Rose Oil Hand Lotion
Invigorating Scrub
Daily Supplements Pack
Cleansing Blend

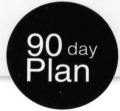

90 day **Plan**

Sleeplessness

Whether you are stressed, sick, struggling with hormones, or depressed, sleeplessness can be hard to overcome, become chronic, and lead to many other health problems. Getting back on track quickly is vital to good health and well-being.

 Our Approach

APPLY *lavender*, *Roman chamomile*, *vetiver,* or *Calming Blend*—start with the scent you like best. You can put it on your wrists, feet, and neck as well as on pillows and bed clothes.

TRY the *Daily Supplements Pack* capsules.

DIFFUSE your favorite calming oil. We like *lavender*, *orange,* or *Calming Blend*.

At Wesleyan University, Connecticut, researchers found that the scent of lavender increased deep, restful sleep for both men and women. But remember, the body responds better to complete darkness. Even the light from an alarm clock can interrupt sleep. Move small lights at least three feet from the bed.

Your Inner Geek

A study published in the journal *Appetite* found "concrete links between particular nutrients and sleep duration in a large survey of adults, studying real-life sleep patterns for a year," says Michael Grandner, a researcher at the University of Pennsylvania's Center for Sleep and Circadian Neurobiology. "Very short sleepers had the narrowest nutrient range, which could mean their sleep-deprived brains are making poor food choices or they're eating the same unhealthy snacks day after day," he explains.

"Very short sleepers also got less lycopene, a nutrient abundant in tomatoes, carrots, bell peppers, and other red and orange foods. As for short sleepers, they lacked vitamin C and selenium, a mineral found in fish, seafood, turkey, and barley."
Men's Journal

"Traditionally, chamomile preparations such as tea and essential oil aromatherapy have

been used to treat insomnia and to induce sedation (calming effects). Chamomile is widely regarded as a mild tranquilizer and sleep-inducer. Sedative effects may be due to the flavonoid, apigenin, that binds to receptors in the brain."
Phytotherapy Research

Integrate

What's troubling you? For most of us when we can't sleep, it is our mind racing about unfinished issues or problems, or we find ourselves worrying because we can't sleep. Even emotional health can contribute to our ability to sleep. Calming your stress can help you sleep soundly. Follow our easy oil and supplement suggestions in the 90-Day Plan Cheat Sheet in the section on Depression, and enjoy a good night's sleep.

Did you know?

Coffee drinkers are far more likely to be poor sleepers. Caffeine and other dietary metabolic disrupters like MSG, sugar, white flour, and other carbohydrates make you think that you are "perking up" in the morning. In truth, they are actually disrupting your ability to sleep at night, even if these foods and drinks are taken only in the morning.

The main reason is their stress on your adrenal glands. In addition, your body's dependence on them will interrupt natural serotonin (the feel-good hormone) production. Without natural serotonin production, we can become sad, grumpy, and depressed. Over time you may find you are not only unable to sleep but experience a dull ache in your lower back. Try taking **Energy & Stamina Complex** instead of caffeine and sugar in the morning. Applying **Detoxification Blend** and **sandalwood** to the lower back can help support the adrenals.

Dive In!

"Cheating Ourselves of Sleep" by Jane E. Brody, *The New York Times*, June 17, 2013.

Healthy Sleep Habits, Happy Child by Marc Weissbluth, One of the country's leading researchers updates his revolutionary approach to solving—and preventing—your children's sleep problems (Paperback, 2003).

Cheat Sheet

MONTH 1
lavender
Daily Supplements Pack
Calming Blend

MONTH 2
Daily Supplements Pack
orange
vetiver

MONTH 3
Daily Supplements Pack
Roman chamomile
Calming Blend

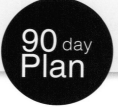

90 day **Plan**

Sore Throat

There are many reasons why sore throats arise. Whether it's post nasal drip from allergies or swelling from a virus or an infection, that familiar pain is one that we all want to get rid of quickly.

Our Approach

APPLY 1–2 drops of *lemon*, *lavender* and/or a *Protective Blend* (diluted) to the outside of the throat. Still have pain? Add 1–3 drops of diluted *Soothing Blend* or *clove* oil on top of the other oils.

TRY *Protective Throat Drops* or *Protective Beadlets* periodically during the day. Add *lemon* or *Protective Blend* to a cup of tea or warm water. You can also try a drop of *lemon* and *frankincense* on the back of the throat. Take the *Daily Supplements Pack* and a *Probiotic Defense Formula* capsule daily.

DIFFUSE *eucalyptus* or *Cleansing Blend* during the day and *lavender* at night.

Our favorite sore throat fighters are **Protective Blend Throat Drops** or a drop of **Protective Blend** on a spoon with honey or another natural sweetener. Also try adding 20 drops of **Protective Blend** to a 2 oz. spray bottle with water to make your own throat spray.

Your Inner Geek

Many people find that a gargle with lemon juice and water, can actually help their sore throat and help make it feel better. The acidic nature of lemon juice can sometimes change the environment and might help chase away some of the viruses (ABC News).

A recent study by a team of surgeons found that a solution made with **cinnamon** oil killed a number of common and hospital-acquired infections, like streptococcus and methicillin-resistant Staphylococcus aureus, or MRSA. The study found it was just as effective as several antiseptics widely used in hospitals. Another study by French researchers in 2008 had similar results, showing that at concentrations of 10 percent or less, **cinnamon** oil was effective against Staphylococcus, E. coli ,and several antibiotic-resistant strains of bacteria (*The New York Times*).

Integrate

Remember to order everything needed for cold and flu season before it starts. Be sure to order from the 90-Day Plan Cheat Sheet in the section on Colds. We like to diffuse year-round to keep germs and toxins at bay. Some oils are more costly than others, so keep the more expensive oils for applying and the less expensive oils for diffusing. Inexpensive **lemon** oil is great for diffusing while it eases a sore throat.

Did you know?

Sore throats can often be the first sign of an illness, and ignoring it will often put you on a longer path to wellness. Providing a humidifier or cool mist diffuser (with essential oils) in your child's bedroom is also helpful in reducing the dry air, which can aggravate any sore throat. Gargling is an excellent way to deal with a sore throat. Try adding essential oils to salt water and gargling with this mixture for as long as you can (Andrew Weil, MD).

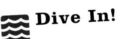

Dive In!

The Tipping Point: How Little Things Can Make a Big Difference by Malcolm Gladwell
Just as a single sick person can start an epidemic of the flu, so too can a small but precisely targeted push cause a fashion trend, the popularity of a new product, or a drop in the crime rate (Paperback, 2002).

To treat a sore throat, few remedies are as tried-and-true as honey. Just make sure you use raw honey, as the vast majority of honey for sale in the United States is highly processed or refined, which, like most other refined foods, can promote disease and damage your health rather than help (Joseph Mercola, MD).

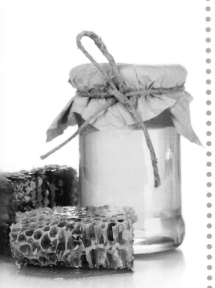

Cheat Sheet

MONTH 1
lavender
lemon
Daily Supplements Pack
Protective Blend
Protective Throat Drops

MONTH 2
Soothing Blend
frankincense
Daily Supplements Pack
Protective Beadlets
Cleansing Blend

MONTH 3
clove
eucalyptus
Daily Supplements Pack
Probiotic Defense Formula

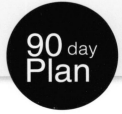

90 day **Plan**

Sports Performance

Most people start an exercise program knowing what equipment to use and even how to dress; but how often do we consider what additional nutrition we may need? Here is a place to start...

Our Approach

APPLY *Soothing Rub* to muscles after bathing to help prevent injury. Our muscles work in groups, and we tend to compensate on one side when the other is weakened; so supporting both sides of the body is key. Applying *peppermint* before activity has been shown to increase performance.

TRY the *Trim Shake* to give your body extra nutrition and to help balance metabolism. Taking the *Daily Supplements Pack* and *Energy & Stamina Complex* twice daily may help to boost your energy level and endurance. A *Peppermint Beadlet* can help to cool you down when exercising in hot weather.

DIFFUSE *peppermint* to increase mental acuity and athletic performance.

Recent studies support that physical performance is seasonal. When vitamin D levels peak due to sun exposure, physical performance peaks as well. Supplements with vitamin D, such as in *Food Nutrient Complex,* can help you to optimize your vitamin D levels even during the long dark months of winter.

Your Inner Geek

There have been a number of studies using Asian ginseng (found in *Energy & Stamina Complex*) for athletic performance in people and laboratory animals. Results have been mixed, with some studies showing better strength and endurance, others showing improved agility or reaction time, and others showing no effect at all. Even so, athletes often take Asian ginseng, which was also found to reduce fatigue in a study of 332 people, to boost both endurance and strength (University of Maryland Center).

Studies suggest that *Withania somnifera* (found in *Energy & Stamina Complex*) may promote growth in children and improve hemoglobin level, red blood cell count, and physical performance in adults (Mishra LC, Singh BB, Dagenais S Altern Med Rev. 2000 Aug; 5(4):334-46).

Integrate

 We've all heard the expression, "No pain, no gain." Pain is our body's way of telling us we are working hard, but it is also our body's signal to either slow down or work smarter. Use healthy supplementation to relieve stress in the body, and be generous with your essential oil use when dealing with injury.

Did you know?

Compounds found in *Energy & Stamina Complex* and the *Daily Supplements Pack* provide powerful nutrition for quick bursts of energy while helping to regulate blood pressure, improve vision, and enhance cardiovascular health—all necessary for peak performance—without the negative side effects of caffeine, sugar, or drugs.

Dive In!

"Help Make Your Body 62% Stronger - Flood it With this Nutrient" by Joseph Mercola, MD, June 15, 2011. A little-known carotenoid called astaxanthin is now believed to be the most potent antioxidant nature has to offer.

Your Best Body Now: Look and Feel Fabulous at Any Age the Eat-Clean Way by Tosca Reno (Paperback 2010).

Cheat Sheet

MONTH 1
Soothing Rub
Daily Supplements Pack
Energy & Stamina Complex
Trim Shake

MONTH 2
Daily Supplements Pack
Energy & Stamina Complex
peppermint
Trim Shake

MONTH 3
Soothing Rub
Daily Supplements Pack
Energy & Stamina Complex
Trim Shake

90 day **Plan**

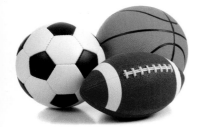

Stress Relief & Relaxation

Daily relaxation is a necessity for good health and to help balance the physical and emotional stresses of life. Over time, stress compounds and can do cumulative damage. The solution is a combination of good nutrition, exercise, and sleep.

 ## Our Approach

APPLY *Tension Blend* to your pulse points. Carry this blend with you, and reapply it as necessary. Alternate with *lavender*, *Grounding Blend,* and *Calming Blend* when stress is severe. Apply *Detoxification Blend* to the lower back to support your adrenals. After an evening shower or bath, apply *Rose Oil Hand Lotion* with a drop or 2 of essential oils to your entire body.

TRY the *Daily Supplements Pack* during the day to keep your daytime energy up so that you can sleep more restfully at night.

DIFFUSE your favorite calming oil. We like *lavender*, *bergamot*, *white fir,* or *Calming Blend*.

White fir
can help to reduce cortisol levels (stress hormones). Apply or diffuse this oil in the morning before you face the world. Take some time to pray or meditate while diffusing. Take a walk and breathe...deeply.

Your Inner Geek

Brazilian scientists had participants spend five minutes inhaling one of three substances: sweet orange essential oil, tea tree oil, or plain water. Participants then underwent a stressful test while having their vital signs measured. Those who sniffed orange oil were less anxious throughout the test, and the beneficial effects even lingered once the exam was over (Prevention.com).

When applying oil formulas, give yourself several minutes of slow, deep, even breathing while you imagine how, with each breath, the oil molecules are entering your bloodstream and spreading throughout your body, relaxing tight muscles and alleviating tensions and strain. These moments will soon become one of your favorite times of the day (*Discovery Fit & Health*).

> **The ability to summon positive emotions during periods of intense stress lies at the heart of effective leadership.—Jim Rohn**

Integrate

 Jump start your stress reduction program by using **Aroma Massage Technique**. Look online for the practitioner nearest you; or get an **Aroma Massage Kit,** and have a friend or family member apply oils to your feet and back.

Did you know?

Busy people often feel anxious, depressed, or exhausted. They also may have short fuses, gain weight easily, or have weak immune systems. These symptoms can often be attributed to one thing: adrenal fatigue. The stress of living in overdrive on a daily basis can burn you out. **Energy & Stamina Complex** can help rejuvenate the energy center of the cell (mitochondria), helping to alleviate emotional and physical fatigue.

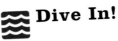 **Dive In!**

"Mental Health: Stress" by Dr. Andrew Weil, MD, drweil. com, July 27, 2013.

The Big Book of Stress Relief Games: Quick, Fun Activities for Feeling Better by Robert Epstein (Paperback 2000).

Cheat Sheet

MONTH 1
Grounding Blend
Daily Supplements Pack
Calming Blend
Detoxification Blend
Trim Shake

MONTH 2
bergamot
lavender
Daily Supplements Pack
Detoxification Blend

MONTH 3
Rose Oil Hand Lotion
Daily Supplements Pack
white fir
Detoxification Blend

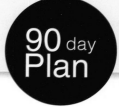

90 day **Plan**

Virus

Viruses, according to the Mayo Clinic are "capsules," smaller than cells, that contain genetic material. To reproduce, viruses invade cells of the body, hijacking the machinery that makes cells work. During this process, host cells are eventually destroyed. Viruses are responsible for everything from AIDS to the common cold, including Ebola virus, hemorrhagic fever, genital herpes, influenza, measles, smallpox, herpes, molluscum, chicken pox, warts, and shingles.

Our Approach

APPLY oils often but in small amounts! Apply 1–2 drops of *melaleuca*, *melissa*, *rosemary*, *oregano*, *sandalwood*, *thyme,* or *Protective Blend* to the bottoms of the feet and along the spine (diluted) every 1–2 hours, or as often as you can.

TRY *Daily Supplements Pack* and *Protective Softgels* every 4 hours (finish the bottle); then take one *Probiotic Defense Formula* capsule a day after that.

DIFFUSE a good germ-fighting oil. Our favorites are *lemon*, *eucalyptus*, *Cleansing Blend*, *Protective Blend,* and *Respiratory Blend*.

Your Inner Geek

A 2008 study examined the antiviral effect of lemon balm oil —the essential oil of *melissa* officinalis—on herpes simplex virus (HSV-1 and 2), finding that higher concentrations of lemon balm oil (*melissa*) abolished viral infectivity nearly completely (Phytomedicine).

If you are not using *Protective* products in your house, now is the time to start. Using them will rob a virus of its strength. Diffuse *Protective Blend*; clean with *Protective Cleaner*: spray on telephones, light switches, and door knobs; and wash hands with *Protective Hand Wash*.

Integrate

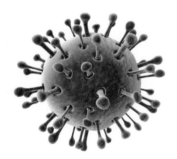

Is taking essential oils with whole food supplements more effective than taking each one alone? Just like a good sauce has many ingredients, good health comes from many sources.

Did you know?

Coconut oil is highly antiviral. Bruce Fife, author of the *The Coconut Oil Miracle , shares*, "Laboratory tests have shown that the MCFAs (medium chain fatty acids) found in coconut oil are effective in destroying viruses that cause influenza, measles, herpes, mononucleosis, hepatitis C and AIDS; bacteria that can cause stomach ulcers, throat infections, pneumonia, sinusitis, urinary tract infections, meningitis, gonorrhea and toxic shock syndrome; fungi and yeast that lead to ringworm, candida and thrush; and parasites that can cause intestinal infections such as giardiasis."

Due to the way it is processed, **coconut oil** has a high concentration of capric acid and caprylic acid, which gives it an amazing amount of antioxidant and disinfecting properties. Mix coconut oil with an essential oil like **oregano** to dilute the heat but maintain the potency.

≋ Dive In!

The Coconut Oil Miracle by Bruce Fife (Paperback 2004).

"Are Viruses Alive?: Although Viruses Challenge Our Concept of What 'Living' Means, They Are Vital Members of the Web of Life" by Luis P. Villarreal, *Scientific American,* August 8, 2008.

Cheat Sheet

MONTH 1
Daily Supplements Pack
melissa
Protective Hand Wash
Protective Softgels
oregano

MONTH 2
melaleuca
Daily Supplements Pack
Protective Blend
Protective Cleaner
Protective Softgels
thyme

MONTH 3
Respiratory Blend
lemon
Daily Supplements Pack
Protective Softgels
Probiotic Defense Formula
Cleansing Blend

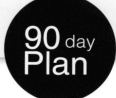

90 day **Plan**

Vision

Vision problems can include changes in eye sight, glaucoma, cataracts, or even macular degeneration. The foods we eat, how we take care of our eyes, and the amount of sleep we get all factor into eye health.

 ## Our Approach

APPLY 1–2 drops of *frankincense*, diluted, around the eyes.

TRY the *Daily Supplements Pack* capsules 1–2 times daily.

DIFFUSE *lavender* or *Calming Blend* to help you sleep at night. A good night's rest is very important for eye health.

Compounds in *frankincense*, including boswellic acid, are very healing to the eyes. Their anti-inflammatory powers and ancient historical uses demonstrate their effective applications in eye health.
Ray Sahelian, MD

Your Inner Geek

 A 2009 study by the National Eye Institute in the United States found that omega-3 fatty acids helped to protect adults from both age-related macular degeneration (AMD) and dry-eye syndrome (Dr. Guillermo Rocha, ophthalmologist and medical director of GRMC Vision Centre in Brandon, Manitoba).

In another study, the antioxidant vitamins C, E, beta carotene, and zinc reduced the risk of developing advanced AMD by about 25%, according the National Eye Institute's original Age-Related Eye Disease Study (AREDS) (Chicago Tribune, May 30, 2012).

Integrate

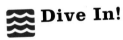 Purchasing pure, therapeutic-grade products is crucial. This grade sets the essential oil apart from all others because all stages of production are carefully monitored and independently tested.

Did you know?

One of the keys to good vision health is carotenoids. Carotenoids are natural pigments that are synthesized by plants and are responsible for the bright colors of various fruits and vegetables. In food, blueberries contain potent antioxidants that support healthy neurological function and aid in normal eye health. Can't eat blueberries every day? The **Daily Supplements Pack** contains powerful carotenoid antioxidant protection from lutein, lycopene, natural alpha and beta carotene, and astaxanthin that support healthy vision.

≋ Dive In!

"Closing in On a Cure for Vision Loss" by Jonathan D. Rockoff, *Wall Street Journal*, July 23, 2012.

Vision and Art: The Biology of Seeing by Margaret S. Livingstone (Hardcover 2008).

Cheat Sheet

MONTH 1
Daily Supplements Pack
frankincense
lavender

MONTH 2
Daily Supplements Pack
frankincense
Calming Blend

MONTH 3
Daily Supplements Pack
frankincense
lavender

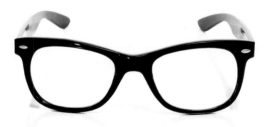

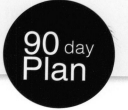

90 day Plan

Weight Management

Culture, age, sex, diet, sleep, stress, exercise, and medications all factor into our ability to manage an ideal weight. With the right approach, everyone can achieve the weight that they desire.

💡 Our Approach

APPLY *peppermint* to the back of your neck to help reduce cravings, and apply *Metabolic Blend* over areas of fat at least twice a day.

TRY taking 5 drops of *Metabolic Blend* in 16 oz. of water or 1–3 drops under the tongue or in a capsule, daily, to help regulate your metabolism. Take *Daily Supplements Pack* and *Digestive Enzyme Complex* capsules daily. Add oils and supplements from the chart in our "Did You Know" section for added benefits. Replace 1–2 meals daily with a vanilla or chocolate *Trim Shake*. Take *Peppermint Beadlets* when cravings strike.

DIFFUSE *Invigorating Blend*: we find that this blend helps to reduce the desire to overeat.

Hungry?
Drink a glass of water with a few drops of a citrus oil like *grapefruit* or *Metabolic Blend*. Most of us are not really hungry, we are thirsty. Fill the void with hydration instead of empty calories. Need something to munch on? Try a water-rich whole food like cucumbers or watermelon.

Your Inner Geek

Naringenin, a flavonoid in grapefruit, balances out blood sugar levels and helps to prevent metabolic syndrome, a pre-diabetic condition associated with weight gain around the waist. Scientists at the University of Western Ontario found it worked by programming the liver to burn up excess fat rather than store it.

According to Cherie Calbom, author of *The Coconut Diet*, replacing your usual cooking oil with coconut oil can aid in weight loss. Coconut fat yields fewer calories per gram than other fats, producing only 6.8 calories per gram rather than 9 calories like most fats. Unlike most other fats, calories in coconut oil act more like carbohydrates, being burned by the liver for immediate energy, according to the *American Journal of Clinical Nutrition*.

> **In two decades I've lost a total of 789 pounds. I should be hanging from a charm bracelet.** —Erma Bombeck

Integrate

 The key to losing fat is incorporating fat-burning foods, supplements, and essential oils into your daily routine. The list on the next page details the information about the oils and supplements that are great fat burners. Adding at least one every time you eat can help you see the pounds start to melt away and the lean you show through!

Did you know?

Top 10 essential oils and supplements to help aid in weight management:

Essential Oils:

- **Black pepper**: helps reduce hunger, creating a feeling of fullness and reducing fat stores.
- **Invigorating Blend**: aids in increasing metabolism and draining the lymphatic system.
- **Cypress**: helps reduce cellulite, increase detoxification, and improve circulation.

  Grapefruit: aids in the breakdown of fats.
- **Cinnamon**: may help to balance blood sugar.
- **Metabolic Blend**: combines ingredients that help to control hunger and increase metabolism.

Supplements:

- **Trim Shake**: increases appetite satisfaction and balances blood sugar.
- **GI Cleansing Formula**: improves digestion and aids in cleansing.
- **Digestive Enzyme Complex**: improves digestion and eliminates toxins from the body
- **Probiotic Defense Formula**: improves digestion and increases the number of calories burned.
- **Detoxification Complex**: helps to balance the thyroid.

Cheat Sheet

MONTH 1
Daily Supplements Pack
Peppermint Beadlets
Metabolic Blend
Digestive Enzyme Complex
Trim Shake

MONTH 2
Invigorating Blend
Daily Supplements Pack
Metabolic Blend
Digestive Enzyme Complex
Trim Shake

MONTH 3
Daily Supplements Pack
peppermint
Metabolic Blend
Digestive Enzyme Complex
Trim Shake

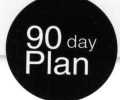

≈ Dive In!

Eat to Live: The Amazing Nutrient-Rich Program for Fast and Sustained Weight Loss by Joel Fuhrman (Paperback, Revised Edition January 5, 2011).

Fast Food Nation: The Dark Side of the All American Meal by Eric Schlosser (Paperback, 2005).

Nutritarian Handbook by Joel Fuhrman MD (Paperback, 2010).

Women's Health

Women face unique health challenges from PMS to menopause, weight changes, childbirth, bone loss, headaches, memory, and more. So much about being a woman is multi-tasking. Keeping stress down and energy high is a winning ticket to any woman's health.

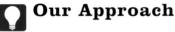 **Our Approach**

APPLY *Women's Monthly Blend* to pulse points, around ankles, or on chest and back when hormone-related symptoms strike. This blend is great for women experiencing PMS or menopausal symptoms.

TRY the *Daily Supplements Pack*, *Bone Nutrient Complex*, and *Phytoestrogen Complex* for nutritional support for your hormones. To help rebuild fallen energy levels, try *Energy & Stamina Complex* daily in place of stimulants like caffeine and sugar.

DIFFUSE *ylang ylang,* or roll on a little *Women's Monthly Blend* in the palm of your hand to inhale when symptoms strike.

Your Inner Geek

 Genistein, a soy-derived isoflavone (found in *Phytoestrogen Complex*), has estrogenic activity and is used as a natural substitute for estrogen replacement therapy in postmenopausal women. Genistein was also shown to decrease fat pad weight in female mice (*The Journal of Nutrition*, 2006). In a separate study, Genistein exhibited antioxidant, antiangiogenic (stops the growth of tumors), and immunosuppressive activities (The National Cancer Institute).

Lowering cortisol by reducing or eliminating coffee and other sources of caffeine can help to improve your skin, hair, and appearance. Begin drinking water with essential oils. Supercharge your day with *Detoxification Complex* and *Phytoestrogen Complex*.

> A woman is like a tea bag—you can't tell how strong she is until you put her in hot water. —Eleanor Roosevelt

Integrate

Hormones can be a tricky business. Symptoms like weight gain, headaches, change in body structure, hair loss, bone loss, lack of energy, and more are often caused by hormone imbalance. Start by getting an accurate blood test to see where your levels are and where they should be for you. Then incorporate supplements and oils to help bring you back into balance.

Did you know?

The biggest challenge to a woman's health is the queen of stress hormones: cortisol. A stress-filled life, lack of sleep, age, environmental and nutritional stresses, lack of exercise, and caffeine can drive cortisol to dangerous levels. Help reduce cortisol levels with **Women's Monthly Blend** and **Phytoestrogen Complex**.

Cortisol also inhibits the growth of beneficial microflora in the intestines. These essential bacteria support the immune system, create B vitamins, and increase the absorption of minerals like calcium, iron, and magnesium. A decrease in their population can result in more colds, sore throats, headaches, diarrhea, upset stomachs, and the overgrowth of harmful bacteria and fungus like candida. Help build healthy intestinal flora with **Probiotic Defense Formula**.

Moodiness, anxiety, depression, and headaches are all consequences of elevated cortisol's long-term effects on serotonin and dopamine production and may even cause brain cells to shrink. Help relieve the symptoms of anxiety and depression with **bergamot** and **Joyful Blend**.

 Dive In!

Women's Bodies, Women's Wisdom by Christiane Northrup, MD (Paperback, 2010).

Mother-Daughter Wisdom: Understanding the Crucial Link Between Mothers, Daughters and Health by Christiane Northrup, MD (Paperback 2006).

Cheat Sheet

MONTH 1
Bone Nutrient Complex
Daily Supplements Pack
Women's Monthly Blend
Phytoestrogen Complex

MONTH 2
Bone Nutrient Complex
Daily Supplements Pack
ylang ylang

MONTH 3
Bone Nutrient Complex
Daily Supplements Pack
Women's Monthly Blend
Phytoestrogen Complex

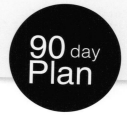

90 day **Plan**

Glossary of Blends & Supplements

Blends

Anti-Aging Blend
Look for a blend with frankincense, sandalwood, lavender, myrrh, helichrysum, or rose

Calming Blend
Look for a blend with lavender, Roman chamomile, sandalwood, sweet marjoram, vanilla, or ylang ylang

Cleansing Blend
Look for a blend with cilantro, citronella, lemon, lime, melaleuca, or pine

Detoxification Blend
Look for a blend with clove, grapefruit, or rosemary

Digestive Blend
Look for a blend with ginger, peppermint, tarragon, fennel, caraway, coriander, or anise

Focus Blend
Look for a blend with amyris, frankincense, lime, patchouli, Roman chamomile, sandalwood, or ylang ylang

Grounding Blend
Look for a blend with spruce, rosewood, frankincense, or blue tansy

Invigorating Blend
Look for a blend with orange, lemon, grapefruit, mandarin, bergamot, or tangerine

Joyful Blend
Look for a blend with tangerine, elemi, lemon myrtle, melissa, ylang ylang, or sandalwood

Massage Blend
Look for a blend with cypress, marjoram, peppermint, basil, grapefruit, or lavender

Metabolic Blend
Look for a blend with grapefruit, lemon peppermint, ginger, or cinnamon

Protective Blend
Look for a blend with cinnamon, clove bud, eucalyptus, rosemary, or orange

Repellent Blend
Look for a blend with citronella

Respiratory Blend
Look for a blend with peppermint, eucalyptus, tea tree, and lemon

Soothing Blend
Look for a blend with wintergreen, camphor, peppermint, blue tansy, blue chamomile, or helichrysum

Tension Blend
Look for a blend with basil, cilantro, frankincense, lavender, marjoram, peppermint, Roman chamomile, rosemary, or wintergreen

Topical Blend
Look for a blend with black cumin seed oil, rosewood, eucalyptus globulus, geranium, lemongrass, or melaleuca

Women's Blend
Look for a blend with bergamot, cinnamon, jasmine absolute, patchouli, rose absolute, sandalwood, vetiver, or ylang ylang

Women's Monthly Blend
Look for a blend with clary sage, lavender, bergamot, Roman chamomile, cedarwood, ylang ylang, or geranium

Supplements

Bone Nutrient Complex
Look for a supplement that combines calcium, magnesium, potassium, and zinc with essential oils

Cellular Vitality Complex
Look for a supplement that will support healthy cell proliferation and lifespan and support healthy cellular inflammatory response

Chewable Multivitamin
Look for a supplement that contains a blend of vitamins A, C, and E and botanical extracts

Daily Supplements Pack
Look for a Daily Supplements Pack that contains an omega-3 supplement, a multivitamin complex, and a cellular energy blend in easy to swallow capsules

Detoxification Complex
Look for a supplement that supports healthy cleansing and filtering functions of the liver, kidneys, colon, lungs, and skin

Digestive Enzyme Complex
Look for a multi-enzyme complex to promote good digestion with peppermint and fennel

Digestive Softgel
Look for a supplement that contains a blend of ginger, peppermint, and tarragon

Energy & Stamina Complex
Look for a supplement that contains a bio-available energy and stamina complex

Essential Oil Cellular Complex
Look for a supplement that contains the essential oils of frankincense, lemongrass, and thyme

Essential Oil Cellular Complex Liquicaps
Look for a supplement in liquicaps form that contains the same healthy antioxidant oils listed in the complex above

Essential Oil Omega Complex
Look for a supplement that contains a clinically-proven dose of omega-3 fatty acids with lemongrass and clove essential oils

Food Nutrient Complex
Look for a supplement that contains a blend of chlorophyll, rich botanicals, choline, and amino acids to boost vitality and reduce stress

GI Cleansing Formula
Look for a supplement that contains the essential oils of oregano and cinnamon that may help to improve the body's immune defenses

Omega-3 Fish Oil
Look for a supplement that contains minerals enhanced with lemon and cinnamon essential oils

Phytoestrogen Complex
Look for a supplement that contains a blend of natural plant extracts that support hormone balance throughout the different phases of a woman's life

Probiotic Defense Formula
Look for a supplement that contains a high-potency probiotic that can help support core intestinal health

Trim Shake
Look for an essential oil–infused superfood meal replacement shake

Vegan Essential Oil Omega Complex
Look for a supplement that is 100% vegan-friendly with natural plant-sourced fatty acids

Index

Index